COMPUTER SCIENCE, TECHNOLOGY AND APPLICATIONS

COMPUTER GRAPHICS

Computer Science, Technology and Applications

Additional books in this series can be found on Nova's website under the Series tab.

Additional E-books in this series can be found on Nova's website under the E-book tab.

COMPUTER SCIENCE, TECHNOLOGY AND APPLICATIONS

COMPUTER GRAPHICS

MARTIN J. DAVIS
EDITOR

Nova Science Publishers, Inc.
New York

For permission to use material from this book please contact us:
Telephone 631-231-7269; Fax 631-231-8175
Web Site: http://www.novapublishers.com

LIBRARY OF CONGRESS CATALOGING-IN-PUBLICATION DATA

Computer graphics / editor, Martin J. Davis.
p. cm.
Includes index.
ISBN 978-1-61761-811-6 (hardcover)
1. Computer graphics. 2. Digital images. 3. Imaging systems in medicine. 4. Information visualization. 5. Computer-aided design. I. Davis, Martin J.
T385.C5584 2011
620'.00420285--dc22
2011006687

Published by Nova Science Publishers, Inc. † New York

CONTENTS

PREFACE

Computer graphics are graphics created using computers and, more generally, the representation and manipulation of image data by a computer. The development of computer graphics, has made computers easier to interact with, and better for understanding and interpreting many types of data. Developments in computer graphics have had a profound impact on many types of media and have revolutionized animation, movies and the video game industry. This book presents current research in the study of computer graphics, including computer graphics and medical image processing utilized in oral and maxillofacial surgery; open-source and freeware tools in computer graphics; fractal geometry in computer graphics and virtual reality; and visual attention in computer graphics.

Chapter 1 - Computer Aided Design (CAD) is a vital application area of the all-pervasive Information Technology Revolution influencing the way we live and work, shrinking the effects of time and distance, and altering the very nature of work in an organization. Modern computers (even a PC) can generate and process information on a scope never before possible. Such information, generated in tables of numbers of hundreds of pages long, may be of no worth to a human user unable to comprehend them, but may be very meaningful if presented graphically. Computer graphics, which is a study of techniques to improve communication between human and machine, is an important component of CAD. Adoption of CAD in various fields has accelerated with recent advances in microcomputer technology, steady decline in cost of computers, and tremendous increase in their computing power and graphic capabilities. This is equally applicable in Architecture (including Planning), Civil-Building Engineering, and Construction (usually classified as A-E-C) field. Real utility of Computer Aided Design (CAD) is not confined to just producing sophisticated solid geometry's or giving more stress to cosmetic such as producing neater, more attractive drawing packages only. It should cover many other aspects of design adopting an Integrated Computer-Aided Design Approach (covering all its components including graphics, drafting, geometric modeling, optimization and so on), involving hundreds of variables, to enhance *Productivity*, *Social-Responsiveness*, and other benefits, particularly in Urban Development and Management, creating scope for informed *public-participation* in the decision-making process in such operations.

The chapter highlights planning and designs as a problem solving process and the vital role of computers and graphics in this process. It outlines the concept of Integrated Computer Aided Design; it's components, and the utility and application of computer graphics in *geometric modeling*, *design analysis*, *design optimization*, and in architectural and engineering drafting. It gives illustrative graphic application results of Integrated Computer Aided Design (ICAD) Software developed by the author for *design analysis* and *design optimization* in integrated computer-aided structural design and drafting, and integrated computer-aided building design and drafting. It presents a case study of *participatory planning and design* using a Descriptive Model in graphic form for urban development planning policy analysis. It gives an example application of graphics programming using AutoLISP for Computer-Aided Design and Drafting (CADD) of urban layout modules. The need for universal graphic standard programming like GKS in the AEC sector is stressed, which will greatly facilitate application of Integrated Computer Aided Design in this sector to derive various benefits including *Efficiency* and *Effectiveness*. To make such applications feasible, a *compulsory* addition of "*Computer Aided Planning and Design by Optimization*", as a full-length *subject of study* (suggestive course-content in Appendix) for the AEC Professional Degree Curriculum, is suggested. This will help equip AEC Professionals, who *commit* huge *Resources* in their Planning and Design *Decisions* enjoining on them an *ethical responsibility* for *efficient* and *equitable* use of *resources* so *committed*, to develop and apply such techniques to discharge their *Accountability* for a *Resource-Efficient* and *Equitable* problem solution in this sector.

Chapter 2 - Digital preoperative planning is increasingly utilized in all fields of orthopaedic surgery. Reported advantages are higher accuracy, and reliability, time saving and digitally manipulating radiographs. On the other hand, high cost and unavailability are important limitations for their use. The authors would like to describe their experience with the use of one famous professional graphics editing programs, Adobe photoshop program, to plan their corrective surgeries in cases with deformities of the lower limbs.

In this work, the authors will describe the use of the Adobe photoshop program to correct a post-traumatic genu varus deformity through high tibial osteotomy. Their demonstrations will be limited to the principles of mechanical axis planning in the frontal plane and thereafter, different forms of valgus producing high tibial osteotomy to correct this post-traumatic varus deformity. The same principles can be used everywhere in a reasonably reproducible way.

The authors' demonstrations will be divided into the following areas:

I. Identify the source of deformity
   1. Mark the centers of hip, knee and ankle joints
   2. Mechanical axis and mechanical axis deviation (MAD)
   3. Joint orientation lines
   4. Joint orientation angles
II. Identify the level of the Center of Rotation of Angulation (CORA)
   1. Tibial mechanical axis planning
   2. Femoral mechanical axis planning
III. Simulating corrective osteotomies
   1. Open wedge osteotomy
   2. Maquet dome osteotomy
   3. Reversed focal dome osteotomy
   4. Closing wedge osteotomy

Chapter 3 - Surgical procedures in the cranio-maxillofacial region require a detailed knowledge of this region's complex anatomy. The limited intraoperative visibility, especially the anatomical intricacies, makes this kind of surgery a demanding procedure. Due to the expanding application of computer technology in medicine, new methods are evolving for medical diagnosis and presurgical planning, and especially for guiding or performing surgical interventions. Nowadays, computer-assisted navigation technology has become almost routine in neurosurgery. However, in the field of oral and maxillofacial surgery, these neurosurgery-oriented navigation systems had to be adapted and the software changed, especially with respect to preoperative planning, where more complicated algorithms in computer graphics and medical image processing are involved.

This study presents an image guided system for oral and maxillofacial surgery, which integrates 3D medical modeling, preoperative surgical planning and intraoperative tracking into a surgical navigation system. With the aid of this system, the precision achieved in the planning phase can be transferred to the operating theatre so that the feasibility and reliability of oral and maxillofacial surgery can be achieved in anatomically complex operation sites. Various algorithms in the field of computer graphics and medical image processing are involved in this system, including DICOM file parsing, image segmentation and 3D-visualization, surface decimation, cutting, collision detection, spatial search and 3D distance computing, volume measurement, spline curve generation, boolean operation, multi(curved)-planar reconstruction, image registration, etc. For each of these algorithms, a set of dynamic link libraries (DLL) were developed using C++, as well as the VTK and ITK via object oriented programming methodology. Therefore, a plug-in evolutive architecture was established, allowing for expandability, accessibility, and maintainability in the authors' system. Benefits of the preoperative planning software, as well as this navigation system, are demonstrated in the clinical cases of oral and maxillofacial surgery, ranging from dental implantology to as far as the treatment of craniofacial malformations and advanced tumours within this anatomically complex region.

Chapter 4 - The diverse nature of the term COMPUTER GRAPHICS can be seen in the high number of keywords associated with it. This paper deals with a topic of increasing relevance, that of the use of computer graphics applications in the process of valuing cultural heritage: identification, records and research, protection, training, conservation and restoration, value and dissemination, management of heritage and new technologies.

Research in the field of cultural heritage has benefited from the evolution of the technology of computer graphics, which has undergone exponential development over the last decades. Today it is possible to undertake research which without the aid of modern computers would imply enormous mathematical effort, or which would simply not be possible.

Some of the examples which can be stated are the ability to obtain *in situ* exact virtual models (VM) of heritage elements, their representation and geo-referenced analysis using Geographical Information Systems (GIS), the techniques of Augmented Reality (AR) in the virtual recreations of cultural sites, or the advanced structural analyses which increase our understanding of techniques in use in ancient times.

As a result, there is much excellent research which studies this cultural heritage, although in many cases the dissemination of the results is partial, and therefore does not fully exploit the educational facet of the research. For example, this is often published in the form of articles, and the multimedia information which is fundamental is lost.

This paper attempts to show how a Learning Management System (LMS) has been used in the recuperation of an example of Industrial Heritage, the *San Francisco* windmill (Véjer de la Frontera, Cádiz, Spain). An open source Content Management System (CMS) is chosen to house the results of the use of Computer Graphics in the field of engineering graphics.

Chapter 5 - The emergence of freeware and open-source software has been unanimously regarded as a technological breakthrough in recent years. Many freeware programs and packages are now widely used by individuals and corporations. Simultaneously, open-source codes are being increasingly incorporated into powerful (not only free but also proprietary) systems and applications. This process is also apparent in computer graphics, where freeware and open-source software is now getting outstanding levels of social and technological acceptance among professional users and companies. In this chapter the authors explore the on-going changes currently happening within the computer graphics community as a consequence of this process. In particular, the chapter discusses some issues related to this new approach, such as the kind of licenses available and their implications for further use. The authors also provide pointers to a large collection of open-source and freeware tools and middleware available to handle just about every development task, briefly emphasizing their potential advantages and drawbacks with respect to their proprietary counterparts. Open-source and freeware tools are described and classified in order to provide their readers with a repository of websites and links where freely-available software can be smoothly downloaded and installed. Some hints to help Their readers to use the appropriate software for specific tasks are also reported.

Chapter 6 - Most would agree that we live in an age characterized by an explosion in data and information. The very rapid increase in computing power often described using Moore's law has enabled scientists, researchers and practitioners to collect, store and analyze unprecedented amounts of data. Tools that enable insights into these large quantities of data are of ever increasing importance.

Chapter 7 - In recent times, Graphics Processing Units (GPUs) are considered not only for graphics, but also for speeding-up the execution of general purpose algorithms that can be expressed following a stream processing model. When GPUs became programmable, the scientific community noticed that the enormous computational power behind these processors could be exploited to accelerate applications in many research fields. As a result, relevant works have been proposed in diverse areas such as computer vision, linear algebra, statistical analysis, physics and biological simulation, database analysis, computational finance and cryptography among others. The first trend on using GPUs to speed-up the execution of general purpose algorithms was somehow tricky, and involved translating algorithms into graphics terms, storing data into textures and invoking rendering operations to perform algorithm computations. In the meantime, GPU architectures have moved to a unified rendering pipeline and have included new hardware resources that can benefit the execution of different kind of applications. Programmability of GPUs has improved and new frameworks like OpenCL are available to combine the power of multi-core CPUs and GPUs in heterogeneous systems. In this chapter a complete review on GPU Computing history, techniques and principles are exposed, together with a deeper insight on the use of GPUs for computer vision and image processing applications. Finally, future trends on GPU and heterogeneous architectures programming are discussed.

Chapter 8 - Fractal geometry is also known as "Mandelbrot's geometry" in honour to its "father" the mathematician Benoit Mandelbrot (b. 1924), that showed how fractals can occur in many different places in mathematics and in other disciplines. Fractal geometry can be used for modelling natural shapes (e.g., fern, trees, seashells, rivers, mountains), and its important applications also appear in computer science, because this "new" geometry permits to compress the images, to reproduce, in the virtual reality environments, the complex patterns and the irregular forms present in nature using simple iterative instructions. The aim of this paper is to present the applications of fractal geometry in computer graphics (to compress images) and in virtual reality (to generate virtual territories and landscapes).

Chapter 9 - The most important aspect of the visual attention is its capacity to rapidly select objects of interest in our visual environment. Objects which are not perceptually important can often go completely unnoticed. In the HVS, the eyes do not scan a scene in a raster-like fashion, but rather they jump so that important parts of the scene fall sequentially onto the fovea, the area of highest visual acuity within our eyes. There are two distinct visual attention processes, which termed bottom-up and top-down. The bottom-up process is purely stimulus driven. This is evolutionary, enabling our eyes to rapidly identify salient information in a scene without volitional control such as a candle burning in a dark room, saturated colors etc. The top-down process is, on the other hand, under voluntary control and enables our visual system to focus on parts of a scene which may be relevant to accomplish a task within that scene. Inattentional blindness is a feature of the HVS which may result in objects in a scene which would normally attract attention, being completely ignored if they are not relevant to the current task.

In: Computer Graphics
Editor: Martin J. Davis

ISBN: 978-1-61761-811-6

Chapter 1

COMPUTER-AIDED DESIGN AND COMPUTER GRAPHICS

B.K.Chakrabarty *

Civil/Structural Engineer & Planner, Ex-HUDCO, New Delhi, India

ABSTRACT

Computer Aided Design (CAD) is a vital application area of the all-pervasive Information Technology Revolution influencing the way we live and work, shrinking the effects of time and distance, and altering the very nature of work in an organization [20,21,27]. Modern computers (even a PC) can generate and process information on a scope never before possible. Such information, generated in tables of numbers of hundreds of pages long, may be of no worth to a human user unable to comprehend them, but may be very meaningful if presented graphically [11, 26, 29, 33,34]. Computer graphics, which is a study of techniques to improve communication between human and machine, is an important component of CAD [11,19,29, 33,34]. Adoption of CAD in various fields has accelerated with recent advances in microcomputer technology, steady decline in cost of computers, and tremendous increase in their computing power and graphic capabilities [11,15,19]. This is equally applicable in Architecture (including Planning), Civil-Building Engineering, and Construction (usually classified as A-E-C) field [11,15,24,29]. Real utility of Computer Aided Design (CAD) is not confined to just producing sophisticated solid geometry's or giving more stress to cosmetic such as producing neater, more attractive drawing packages only [11,15,19,29]. It should cover many other aspects of design adopting an Integrated Computer-Aided Design Approach (covering all its components including graphics, drafting, geometric modeling, optimization and so on), involving hundreds of variables, to enhance *Productivity*, *Social-Responsiveness*, and other benefits, particularly in Urban Development and Management, creating scope for informed *public-participation* in the decision-making process in such operations [9,10,19,21, 29].

The chapter highlights planning and designs as a problem solving process and the vital role of computers and graphics in this process. It outlines the concept of Integrated Computer Aided Design; it's components, and the utility and application of computer

* Corresponding author: e-mail: bibhutichakrabarty@yahoo.co.in), (Tel-91-011-26520564.

graphics in *geometric modeling*, *design analysis*, *design optimization* [1], and in architectural and engineering drafting. It gives illustrative graphic application results of Integrated Computer Aided Design (ICAD) Software developed by the author for *design analysis* and *design optimization* in integrated computer-aided structural design and drafting, and integrated computer-aided building design and drafting [2-10]. It presents a case study of *participatory planning and design* using a Descriptive Model in graphic form for urban development planning policy analysis. It gives an example application of graphics programming using AutoLISP for Computer-Aided Design and Drafting (CADD) of urban layout modules. The need for universal graphic standard programming like GKS [11,19,34] in the AEC sector is stressed, which will greatly facilitate application of Integrated Computer Aided Design in this sector to derive various benefits including *Efficiency* and *Effectiveness*. To make such applications feasible, a *compulsory* addition of "*Computer Aided Planning and Design by Optimization*", as a full-length *subject of study* (suggestive course-content in Appendix) for the AEC Professional Degree Curriculum, is suggested. This will help equip AEC Professionals, who *commit* huge *Resources* in their Planning and Design *Decisions* enjoining on them an *ethical responsibility* for *efficient* and *equitable* use of *resources* so *committed*, to develop and apply such techniques to discharge their *Accountability* for a *Resource-Efficient* and *Equitable* problem solution in this sector.

1. Introduction

In recent years, there is tremendous increase in capabilities of computer hardware's and graphics. As a result there are unparalleled transformations in computers in terms of their capacity to capture data, to analyse, manipulate and store them, to disseminate and communicate information's, and to apply these capabilities in different areas and fields of specialization. Such transformations are occurring with increasing rapidity and frequency in many areas and the rate at which Information Technology (IT) and Computer Applications are spreading to various sectors is truly extraordinary and has few, if any, parallels in technological history. The pervasiveness and cheapness of IT is influencing the way we live, work and enjoys ourselves. Today, information technology and computer application is everywhere shrinking the effects of time and distance and altering the very nature of work in an organization. Many writers view it as the second Industrial Revolution.

In the above process Computer Graphics is playing a very vital role. As mentioned above modern computers (even a PC) can generate and process information on a scope never before possible. Such information, generated in tables of numbers of hundreds of pages long, may be of no worth to a human user unable to comprehend them, but may be very meaningful if presented graphically, and computer graphics is the study of such techniques to improve communication between human and machine [11]. Moreover, Computer Graphics is of great help to make computers extremely 'user-friendly' from the outset where computer can be accessed directly in 'user' language, permitting even lay public users without any computer literacy to use it effectively and meaningfully.

Computer Aided Design (CAD) is a vital application area of the all-pervasive Information Technology Revolution influencing the way we live and work [20,21,27]. Computer graphics is an important component of CAD [11,19,29, 33,34]. Adoption of CAD in various fields has accelerated with recent advances in microcomputer technology, steady decline in cost of computers, and tremendous increase in their computing power and graphic capabilities [11,15,19,29]. This is equally applicable in Architecture (including Planning), Civil-Building Engineering, and Construction (usually classified as A-E-C) field [11,15,24,29]. As a result of recent advances in microcomputer technology, computer-assisted design analysis, optimization and graphics are no longer a luxury enjoyed by only a few large companies that can afford mainframe computers and peripherals. Engineers, Architects, Planners and Urban Managers everywhere have now access to better and cheaper computer hardware and software to produce sophisticated computer analysis, optimization, graphics and drafting. The capabilities of computer hardware and graphics are increasing so rapidly that software engineers in various fields are constantly finding new applications of this technology in various aspects of design work. Computers are also playing a significant role in addressing various social, environmental and development issues for a just society with informed public participation in the decision-making process on such issues, which is very relevant in AEC. Again, in this process Computer Graphics can be of great help to make computers extremely 'user-friendly' from the outset where computer is accessed directly in 'user' language, permitting even lay public users without any computer literacy to participate in the decision-making process on such issues.

Real utility of Computer Aided Design (CAD) is no longer confined to just producing sophisticated solid geometry's and more attractive drawing packages only, but can cover many other aspects of design work including optimization to improve productivity and derive other benefits at various operation levels. To gain such advantages, the pace at which Information Technology and CAD are being adopted by various sectors of industry and professional disciplines, using ever increasing computing power, is truly extraordinary compared to any other technology developed in the past. This is equally applicable in Architecture (including Planning), Civil/Building Engineering & Construction (A-E-C) field, where even now more stress is given to cosmetic such as producing neater, more attractive drawing packages only, instead of adopting an Integrated Computer-Aided Design Approach (covering all its components including Optimization), involving hundreds of variables, to improve Productivity and derive other benefits, particularly in Urban Development and Management.

The purpose of this chapter is to provide to readers, students (future A-E-C professionals), and to practicing professionals, an outline of Computer Aided Design (CAD) as a vital application area of IT, an overview of Integrated CAD in A-E-C sector in the context of ongoing IT Revolution, and the highly critical role and profound utility of computer graphics in this process. It highlights planning and design as a problem solving process involving iteration and evaluation of numerous solutions, being function of numerous variables, making use of computer and CAD indispensable in any field. Utility of computer graphics in various components of Integrated CAD is outlined with illustrative examples of computer graphics in some of these components. It gives some graphic application results of Integrated Computer Aided Design (ICAD) Software developed by the author for *design analysis* and *design optimisation* in integrated computer-aided structural design and drafting, and integrated computer-aided building design and drafting [2-10]. A case study of *participatory planning and design* using a Descriptive Model in graphic form for urban development planning policy analysis, and an example application of graphics programming using AutoLISP for Computer-Aided Design and Drafting (CADD) of urban layout modules, are also presented.

The need for universal graphic standard programming like GKS [11,19,34] in the AEC sector is stressed, which will greatly facilitate application of Integrated Computer Aided Design in this sector to derive various benefits including *Efficiency* and *Effectiveness*. To make such applications feasible, a *compulsory* addition of "*Computer Aided Planning and Design by Optimization*", as a full-length *subject of study* (a suggestive course-content is presented in Appendix) for the AEC Professional Degree Curriculum, is suggested. This will help equip AEC Professionals, who *commit* huge *Resources* in their Planning and Design *Decisions*, to develop and apply such techniques to discharge their *Accountability* for a *Resource-Efficient* and *Equitable* problem solution in this sector.

2. IT Revolution and CAD as an Important IT-Application Area

IT can be considered as the means by which we collect, store, process, and use information. Collection, generation, communication, recording, manipulation, and exploitation of information's are an essential activity in solution of most problems. Hence, use of Computers and IT is essential in all activities (including AEC activities) to help effective problem solution in the respective area. It is built around the scientific, technological, engineering, and management disciplines used in information handling and processing. Engineering production and production management are concerned with the effective use of people, products, plant and processes in modern manufacturing industry. This, in turn, is achieved by the proper selection and implementation of policies and plans involving many factors, which interact with each other. In view of this operational complexity involving information handling and processing, IT is in use in engineering production and production management for many years and several of the basic ingredients of IT predate the present microelectronic revolution. IT also assists the introduction of an *Integrated Systems Approach* to such complex problem solving in modern manufacturing industry, which makes IT such a potentially powerful production management tool. As a result IT and computer application is essential part of the processes internal to most manufacturing/ service organizations, to product design processes, to delivery of services, and to inter-organizational relations. There are many application areas of IT, which is expanding continuously with new developments in IT, and Computer Aided Design (CAD) is an important application area of Information Technology (**IT**)[27].

In the above context it is necessary to study the implications of the all-pervasive Information Technology Revolution, influencing the way we live and work, for one major sector of society- those planning and designing in Architecture, Civil/Building Engineering & Construction (usually classified as AEC field) and those managing at various levels in both commercial and public urban organizations. Clearly, such organizations are dependent on their various environments – for resources, markets, *social legitimacy*, and so on. So the implications of Information Technology (IT) for Architecture, Civil/Building Engineering & Construction management are to some extent inseparable from the broader effects on society. At the level of enterprise strategy, the managerial concern is essentially with the *social legitimacy* of the organization and its role in society, in the light of the uncontrollable and sociopolitical aspects of escalating environmental turbulence taking place due to IT revolution. For the firm it has meant a change from a familiar world of marketing and production to an unfamiliar world of strange technologies, strange competitors, new consumer attitudes, new dimensions of social control and, above all, a questioning of the firm's role in society' [27]. Although, this view is expressed with regard to strategic management related to business policy and planning in general, it is equally applicable in respect of the disciplines of Architecture, Civil/Building Engineering & Construction management and both commercial and public urban organizations.

In recent times there has been a considerable movement towards the direct involvement of the public in the definition of their physical environment with increased sense of social responsibility when a new feeling of community consciousness started prevailing in many low income urban neighbourhoods [30]. People need to participate in the creation of their environment with a feeling of control, which is the only way that their needs and values can be taken into consideration. The ongoing IT Revolution has created tremendous scope for introduction of the users in the decision-making process (i.e. *participation*) but this would require designers to add new capacities to their conventional experience and skills. It is well known that all problem solution in the AEC sector involves collection, generation, communication, recording, manipulation, and exploitation of information, and therefore, use of Computers and IT is essential in AEC activities to help effective problem solution. The current IT revolution and computer graphics capabilities permits computers to be 'user friendly' from outset allowing all professionals, and even lay people/citizens to access computers directly in 'user' language, in which dialogues relates directly to the relevant knowledge base or 'user' priority and concerns (e.g. urban sector). This is of special importance in problem solution in AEC sector, where IT application areas of Computer Aided Planning (CAP) and Computer Aided Design (CAD) can play very important role. Hence, it is essential that designers in AEC sector add capacities like IT-CAD expertise to their conventional knowledge to help the above process.

In the above context AEC/urban sector by not applying IT-CAD and other IT innovations in their various activities cannot remain immune to the revolutionary effects of IT on the work organizations and its members, if the sector/disciplines have to make useful contributions to the all-round development of a country/ society, and also remain relevant in the society without adversely affecting their "social legitimacy". As cited above implications/impact of IT on sector/organizations/entities/ disciplines is inseparable from the broader effects on society and social legitimacy of sector/organizations/ entities/disciplines, and therefore, by not applying IT-CAD and other IT-innovations AEC sector and its disciplines may be instrumental in adversely affecting their "social legitimacy". One of the important steps towards this direction (and one of the urgent actions towards such efforts) could be introduction of individual courses for compulsory and comprehensive Education on CAD (a vital application area of IT but rare in AEC sector in many countries), in various disciplines in AEC sector, and also promoting Research and Development activities in this emerging area, to help equip them to develop and apply IT techniques and tools in their operations.

As mentioned above there are unparalleled transformations in computers in terms of their capacity to capture data, to analyze, manipulate and store them, to disseminate and communicate information's, and to apply these capabilities in different areas and fields of specialization. Such transformations are occurring with increasing rapidity and frequency in many areas and the rate at which IT and Computer Applications are spreading to various sectors is truly extraordinary. Today, information technology and computer application is everywhere shrinking the effects of time and distance and this second Industrial Revolution is altering the very nature of work in an organization including AEC organizations. Again, pervasiveness and cheapness of IT is influencing the way we live, work and enjoys ourselves and is generating a wide range of fundamental questions in all sectors of society needing urgent answers [26]. As outlined above many sectors of society and knowledge disciplines have already initiated actions for adequate response to this new challenge. However, knowledge disciplines of Architectural (including Planning) Engineering-Civil/Building Engineering & Construction (usually classified as AEC) in many countries are slow to initiate vigorous and comprehensive actions for adequate response to this new challenge, at the least by introducing compulsory and comprehensive CAD (a vital application area of Information Technology) instructions covering all its components including Optimization in Architectural/Civil-Building Engineering Schools particularly in the developing countries.

The author feels that such actions are essential if the above *disciplines* have to remain relevant in the society by contributing to the *Effective* and *Efficient* solution of societal problems in the AEC sector, and thus, retain their *social legitimacy* in the above changed context For example application of IT-CAD in *Building Economics* covering development of economic performance measures of interest to developers, owners, contractors, and users; linking Cost Engineering including cost indices, elemental estimating, computerized information systems and model building could be very useful tool for economic analyses of projects both for single buildings, and building components leading to much more *Effective* and *Efficient* solution of such societal problems. Similarly, *Computer-Aided Building Design* including *Optimization* covering Building Engineering design process, methodology, identification of objectives, building codes, formulation of design problems, development and evaluation of design alternatives: conceptual building design: spatial requirements, design of space layout; preliminary building design and synthesis, and performance evaluation using modeling, sensitivity analysis and cost estimation using computer-aided design tools could lead to much more *Effective* and *Efficient* solution of such societal problems. In all these processes computer graphics would play a very vital role. Lack of necessary hardware, software and appropriate courses of instruction and textbooks, covering different topics/ components of CAD relevant to Architectural and Civil/Building Engineering Design, are some of the inhibiting factors affecting above CAD instruction/application. Steady decline in the cost of computers has now made such hardware's affordable even to the smallest Architectural & Civil/ Building Engineering Schools/Offices. Other deficiencies like development of sophisticated software's making best use of modern graphics, and lack of appropriate courses of instruction and textbooks, covering different topics/ components of CAD relevant to Architectural and Civil/Building Engineering Design, needs to be adequately addressed.

3. PLANNING AND DESIGN AS A PROBLEM SOLVING PROCESS AND VITAL ROLE OF COMPUTERS WITH GRAPHICS CAPABILITIES

Planning and Design in Architecture, Planning, Civil Engineering (say, Building/ Housing/Urban Services consuming huge *Resources* and affecting the *quality of life* of people) needs to be viewed as a *problem solving process* involving *search* through *numerous* potential solutions (because of *numerous* design variables involved) to select a particular solution that meets a specified criteria or *goal* (say, *Resource-Efficient* and affordable shelter and urban services design). This makes computer-use indispensable for problem solution in all branches of AEC including architecture and civil engineering, particularly in the context of *search* through *numerous* potential solutions with large variations in *resource-efficiency* indicators, requiring a comprehensive planning and design analysis. This view for planning and design in Architecture, Planning, Civil Engineering/ Urban Development is quite relevant especially in less developed countries to achieve the national *goals* of providing adequate shelter and urban services for all, within the affordability and *Resource-Constraints* at the individual, local, and national level. With increasing population and dwindling per capita *Resources*, this view is equally applicable even in the developed countries, as *we live in a Finite Earth with Finite Resources.*

If the goal is to obtain something that is as yet non-existent, such as the design for a building then the question of how potential solutions may be produced arises, which is answered by constructing a *generative system* to produce a variety of potential solutions [24]. There can be different categories of generative systems to represent potential solutions to a design problem. Symbolic generative systems represent potential solutions by means of symbols such as mathematical equations and design variables, which can take different values to represent a particular design proposal. A computer program (like Software's discussed below) to model a design can constitute a *generative system.* Data structures describing a building design might consist of many hundreds of variables including graphic data, making computer-use indispensable to store, retrieve and operate on such data with great speed. Thus, a design problem can be characterized in terms of *data structures*, *constraints*, *objectives* and a *solution generation procedure* to produce potential solutions for consideration, and a computer can be used in the design process to *store and retrieve data* describing a design, to *test potential solutions* for membership of the goal set, and to *automatically generate solutions* to well defined problems [24]. To store and retrieve data describing a design, a computer performs as a data processing machine to retrieve information's *efficiently* and to generate alphanumeric or graphic displays with great speed replacing and augmenting conventional manual drawings, drafting, specifications writing and so on, improving *productivity.* When computer is utilized to automatically generate solutions it executes a program, which operates upon the data structure to compute and assign particular values to variables, and thus, in this case computer is used as an automated design synthesis machine, and it augments some of the traditional functions of the designers. As cited above AEC Operations (e.g. Building, Housing, Urban Development and so on) consume large *Resources* involving many variables giving numerous solutions with large variations in *resource-efficiency* indicators, *search* of optimal solution becomes quite complex, necessitating use of computers to automatically generate optimal solutions adopting the above procedure.

However, this will need powerful computers with graphic capabilities, which are now readily available.

In the context of architectural design, Mitchell (1977) pointed out that the ability to *integrate* sophisticated analysis and *optimisation* techniques into the *design process* would make it possible to maintain much more *effective cost control* and response to the complex design constraints exploring more alternatives, making people to demand them, and agencies not able to provide them would find it difficult to compete. This is equally applicable in all design problems in the AEC operations. In fact it is imperative to develop Integrated Computer-Aided Design (Integrated CAD) System in different branches of AEC including civil engineering (counting building, housing and urban development) incorporating all the five components Integrated CAD (discussed below) and apply such design tools to derive benefits of productivity and equity in our AEC Operations (such as building, housing and urban development) in this New Millennium.

Utility of computer oriented methods for solving civil engineering problems was accepted long time back emphasizing the urgency for recognition of this necessity by the researchers, analysts and practicing engineers in their service to the civil engineering profession. But, compulsory and comprehensive CAD (a vital application area of Information Technology) instructions covering all its components including Optimisation is very rare in Civil-Building Engineering and Architectural Schools particularly in the developing countries. Again, the concept of Integrated CAD by Optimisation is still not part of professional education curricula in most of our AEC educational institutions inhibiting development and application of such modern techniques in actual professional practice. Sporadic attempts are made by some institutions to include CAD subject related to individual fields like structural engineering. But, resource use in such individual parts is much less compared to the larger systems like housing-urban-development systems, formed by such parts. It is desirable that Civil-Building Engineering and Architectural Schools correct this situation by taking more active role in research, development, and compulsory and comprehensive CAD instructions covering all its components including Optimisation, so that application of such comprehensive and Integrated CAD in the housing and urban development process becomes a standard practice to attain a *resource-efficient* and *equitable* problem solution in such operations, and thus, AEC professionals enhance their professional contribution in achieving the national *goals* of providing adequate shelter and urban services to all, within the affordability and resource-constraints at various levels.

Optimization is a human trait that is as old as antiquity. Even the *ancients*, who had little *technology* and *resource-constraints/population pressure*, applied *Optimization* and perceived that a circle has the greatest ratio of area to perimeter, which is the reason that many ancient cities are circular to minimize the length of city walls to enclose the city's fixed area [1, 20]. On the same analogy modern urban-built-form need to be optimized considering the cost/availability of land and the structural feasibility/cost, where civil engineers have to take a leading role. It is unfortunate that in spite of availability of modern highly powerful computers/graphic systems, such *Optimization* is rarely applied in our modern urban operations, causing a mismatch between land price and built-form and creating many *inequities* and *inefficiencies* and the consequent urban problems (e.g. proliferation of slums, inadequate housing/urban services, environmental degradation and so on, in many countries), which needs urgent correction.

Moreover, AEC professionals belonging to Architecture, Planning, Civil/Building Engineering disciplines *COMMIT* huge *Resources* (land, money, materials etc.) in their Planning and Design Decisions related to building, housing, urban development, and construction operations, making them *Accountable* to achieve *Productivity* (*i.e. efficiency & effectiveness*) and *Equity* in use of *Resources* so committed by them in their Decisions. *Operations Research/Optimisation* and *Computer-Aided Design* (CAD) are *Basic Integrative Techniques* to improve *Productivity* [21,22]. Hence, it is *Basic* that AEC professionals apply such *Techniques* to discharge their above *Responsibility*, for a *Resource-Efficient* and *Equitable* solution of our mounting housing and urban problems in the context of *Resource* and affordability *Constraints* at various levels. Availability of modern computers with tremendous computing and graphic capabilities makes it much easier to apply such *Techniques* in this New Millennium.

Again, the ongoing IT revolution has created considerable scope for direct involvement of the public in the definition and creation of their physical environment with increased sense of social responsibility and a feeling of control and community consciousness in many low income urban neighbourhoods. Moreover, participation is a means of protecting the interests of groups of people as well as of individuals, because it satisfies their needs, but these are very often totally or partially ignored by organizations, institutions, bureaucracies, and the 'expert' planners and designers [30]. To facilitate introduction of the users in the decision-making process (i.e. *participation*) designers have to add new capacities to their conventional experience and skills [30]. Hence, it is essential that designers in AEC sector add capacities like IT-CAD expertise to their conventional knowledge to help the above process as mentioned earlier.

Towards such capabilities author has developed a number of descriptive/*optimizing models* for housing and urban development planning and design that are being transformed to an Integrated CAD System i.e. Application CAD Software: HudCAD [10]. Similarly, *optimising models* for structural design (reinforced concrete beam) are also developed and published elsewhere which are also being converted to Integrated CAD Application Software. In view of utility of Graphics in CAD, particularly to make computers to be 'user friendly' from outset facilitating a participatory planning and design process, Computer Graphics is a very important component in this Integrated CAD System. Some application results, highlighting crucial need of such design techniques and graphic capabilities to achieve a resource-efficient and equitable problem solution with people's participation in AEC operations, are presented later.

4. Utility of Computer Graphics in CAD Pertinent to AEC Sector

As already mentioned we are witnessing an information technology revolution with tremendous growth and development of computer technologies and applications enabling us to generate, collect, store and process information on a scale never before possible. Such information's if properly processed and efficiently and effectively transferred by the computer to human, would greatly help us make decisions, to understand our world and to control its operations, affecting the way we live, work and enjoy ourselves. But, as the volume of information increases efficient and effective transfer of such information from machine to human becomes extremely difficult. For example, a computer can easily generate tables of numbers of hundreds of pages but, such a printout may be of no worth to a reader unable to comprehend it because of its sheer volume consuming enormous time, effecting both efficiency and effectiveness of the process. Computer graphics, which is a study of techniques to improve communication between human and machine, hits this problem directly [34]. Thus, a graph may replace the huge table of numbers and enable the reader to comprehend the relevant patterns and characteristics of the data at a glance, allowing the reader to use such information effectively. Therefore, a computer with graphics capabilities enabling it to express its data in pictorial or graphic form using graphical output devices greatly enhances its ability to provide information to the human user. Such communication can also be a two-way process permitting to input graphical information to the computer using graphical input devices. Since computer-aided planning and design is an iterative process it is often desirable to have the input in alphanumeric or graphic form from the user to alter the output from the computer, and thus, a dialogue can be established through the graphics medium i.e. interactive graphics allowing the user to interact with the machine to get the output design as per requirement. This is discussed in more details and illustrated with planning and design example problems later. Thus, computer graphics make possible communication through pictures, charts, and diagrams, offering a vital alternative to the typewriter's string of symbols, and making communication much more meaningful and participative. Using computer graphics and virtual reality techniques we can walk through a building or urban facility, which is yet to be built, giving vital information's, and input (in much less cost compared to physical modeling or prototype construction) to achieve a better planning and design in AEC sector.

There are many unique capabilities of CAD compared to the conventional traditional design methods, which can be attributed to computer graphics, particularly because of tremendous development in this technology in recent times. Graphics has been an increasingly extensive and important area of computer application and is an important component of CAD to generate graphic portrayal of objects with complex geometries for better appreciation of geometric properties and arrangement of spaces in the designed objects. An application closely related to computer graphics which is helpful in planning and design, is *image processing* that is computer analysis of photographs and other visual materials. Typical applications of *image processing* technology include remote sensing and analysis of earth satellite photographs to extract data about crops, atmospheric and water pollution, mineral deposits, land use, etc. which are very useful data for efficient and effective urban planning and management in the context of urban dynamics. Computer graphics in the form of computer animation of scenes in perspectives is very useful in CAD as it allows sophisticated simulations of movements through an environment to be produced. Real-time visual simulation using a colour television screen has been applied in the simulation of aircraft and spacecraft landing and ship docking. CAD has the unique capability to animate sequences of events on a graphical screen, which is of great value to the designer for evaluating moving objects in simulation studies and in urban traffic control [11,19]. For example, before a decision is taken on final design and implementation, a real life operation of an urban facility could be simulated using such CAD and Virtual Reality Technique (which is not possible in conventional planning and design methods), for better appreciation of the design by all stakeholders. Thus, there is lot of utility of computer graphics in CAD. Some of these unique capabilities, which are very relevant to AEC Design, are outlined in more details below.

4.1. Interactive Computer Graphics and Geometric Modelling in AEC CAD

Newman et al define a graphic system as any collection of hardware and software designed to make it easier to use graphic input and output in computer program [26]. Computer graphics may be static or dynamic. By means of interactive graphics the geometry of the object could be changed by simple commands to the computer to find an acceptable solution. Geometric modeling, defines an object in terms of geometric properties and arrangement of spaces. Thus, characteristic applications of computer graphics techniques include engineering and architectural drafting, production of perspectives, and mapping, while computer graphics and geometric modeling is an essential component of computer-aided design in various fields, which is equally applicable for the AEC sector.

Interactive Computer Graphics in CAD can provide real-time or "instantaneous" communication between the computer and the designer or operator, allowing sketching and drawing to be both input to and output from the computer, offering the operator much more freedom over the traditional input methods that use the keyboard. It enhances the designer's visual appreciation of the component's geometry and also permits the designer to identify obvious errors prompting immediate action by the designer to rectify these errors by adjusting proper design parameters. At the initial or conceptual design stage, the shape of a facility could be represented graphically on a monitor screen even using a computer mouse. This can be converted into a proper two-dimensional or three-dimensional Geometric Model and linked to appropriate numerical analysis models for planning and design analysis and optimization to derive its final shape fulfilling the prescribed requirements. The geometric model can then be used as input to an automated drafting system to produce architectural, planning and engineering drawings.

CAD can demonstrate graphically the complex geometries of a designed object and thus, facilitating better appreciation of the object geometry. In this method the designer and other stakeholders can observe the designed object from selected views with perspectives (e.g. isometric views) to judge its acceptability, and any modification of the geometry (whether two or three dimensional) can be achieved in an interactive manner by simple commands to the computer (by all stakeholders) taking hardly any time. Thus, use of CAD can obviate the need of making prototype solid three-dimensional design models (taking lot of time and resources), which are generally prepared in conventional design methods to help better understanding of the object geometry and its geometric properties.

As earlier mentioned, the IT revolution permits better two-way communication, consultation and even co-determination both directly and indirectly, and the user-citizens/individual stakeholders can be involved directly, or his representative's access to the system can be facilitated, for more satisfying *participative design-decision-making*. Thus, if a system is created, say a *planning/design proposal* (both in alpha-numeric and graphic version), various participative subunits and the interested user citizens could be on-line with each other to give input for a satisfying optimal solution of an urban problem in a given context. This is not possible by conventional manual design methods, but using CAD technique such an objective can be easily achieved.

Geometric modelling defines an object/facility in terms of its geometric properties and arrangement of spaces. Geometric properties such as geometric patterns (and size of independent variables if no size optimisation is desired) indicating the relationship between different components of the object/facility are essential input for subsequent design analysis and optimisation operations. A geometric model can be created by a designer on the monitor screen using the mouse or can be constructed using graphic primitives such as dots, lines, arcs, and curves in case of two-dimensional models. Three-dimensional models can be produced by turnkey systems.

The use of computer graphics and particularly the Interactive Computer Graphics and Geometric Modelling in the Planning and Design Analysis, Design Optimisation, Architectural and Engineering Drafting, Participatory Planning and Design, and in Integrated Computer Aided Design is illustrated below with example problems related to AEC sector.

4.2. Computer Aided Planning and Design Analysis Using Graphics

As earlier mentioned Planning and Design Analysis is the most important part of the whole planning and design process, and generally has two components namely: (1) planning, architectural, and engineering analysis, and may include strength analysis, cost analysis, specific performance analysis and so on, (2) interactive graphics. Such analysis is performed on the conceptual or initial geometry of the facility, making liberal use of geometric modelling, to ensure that not only the facility will satisfy the specified objectives, conditions and criteria (say compliance with space requirements, resource-constraints and cost-affordability) but also is feasible in terms of technical (say satisfaction of planning, architectural, and engineering norms and regulations, satisfaction of structural soundness, based on relevant codes of practice, and so on), financial (say cost-effectiveness based on local/national context), and social conditions as may be applicable (say cost affordability by the intended target group for an urban facility, based on local/ national context and policy analysis). Analytical results can be derived from planning and design codes and regulations, mathematical modelling, and model analysis. The utility of computer graphics in computer-aided planning and design analysis is illustrated below with some examples.

4.2.1. Urban Development Planning Policy Analysis - A Descriptive Numeric-Graphic Model

In conventional urban development practice a Planning Regulation: 'Floor Area Ratio (FAR)', which is also called 'Floor Space Index (FSI)', is specified to achieve *public-welfare* and other objectives in Built-Environment [16, 17, 32]. A Schematic Urban-Built-Form in graphic form is shown in Figure 1 below. A Descriptive-Model of the urban built-form, giving the scientific relationship between FAR (or, FSI) and elements of Urban Built-Form, such as: BU (Built-Unit i.e. dwelling unit, commercial unit and so on), BUS (Built Unit Space i.e. average space per BU), SPO (Semi-Public Open Space i.e. average open-to-sky space per BU), BR (Building Rise i.e. number of floors in Built-Form), BUD (Built Unit Density i.e.

number of BU's per unit area), and GCR (Ground Coverage Ratio), could be expressed as follows [9,10]:

$$FAR = \frac{BUS * BR}{BUS + BR * SPO} \qquad (1)$$

$$BUD = \frac{FAR}{BUS} \qquad (2)$$

$$GCR = \frac{FAR}{BR} \qquad (3)$$

The above scientific relationships apply in any type of building and urban development i.e. residential, commercial and so on, for any size of the planning and development area and could also incorporate Built-Unit-Cost. These expressions, showing a *nonlinear* relationship between some Built-Form-Elements, can be used in "*what-if* studies", *'sensitivity-analysis'* in terms of both *numeric* and *graphic* parameters, and to determine the *'Interaction'* between selected built-form-elements to develop an *insight* into their inter-relationships including Costs, for *rational decision making* by the *Planner* and *Designer*. These mathematical equations could also be used to develop *Optimizing Models* (both LCO and MBO Models) for Urban-Built-Form presented later.

The Software Module "CAUB/CADUB" of "HudCAD" uses such scientific relationships including costs and the *Optimizing Models*. Using the above Numeric-Graphic Descriptive-Model and the Software "CAUB/CADUB" the sensitivity of Built-Unit-Cost to the Floor Area Ratio could be instantly depicted in alphanumeric terms as shown in Table-1 below.

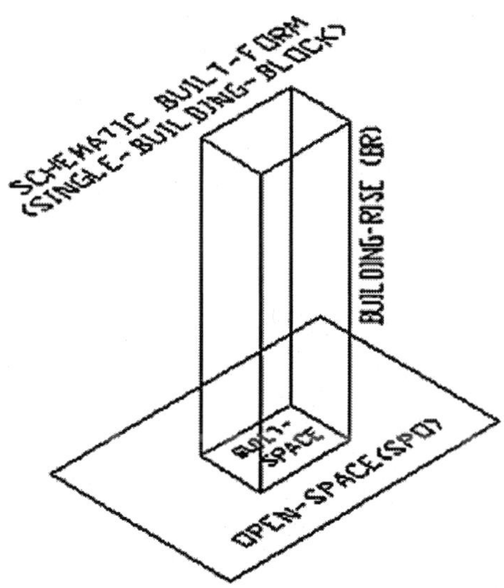

Figure 1. Shematic Urban-Built-Form (Single Building Block).

Table 1. Sensitivity of Cost per Built-Unit (BUC) to the Floor Area Ratio (FAR)

Floor Area Ratio (FAR)	Cost per Built-Unit (BUC) (Monetary Unit or MU)
0.50	2697722
0.83	1825140
1.16	1450552
1.49	1243371
1.82	1112860
2.15	1024101
2.48	960905
2.81	914899
3.14	881542
3.47	858540
3.80	845330
4.13	843416
4.46	858390
4.79	908318
5.12	1076664
5.45	3664320

Some Input-Values Chosen in the above Case are:
BUS= 110.00 Sq.M. SPO= 20.0 Sq.M. LP= 10000 MU/Sq.M.

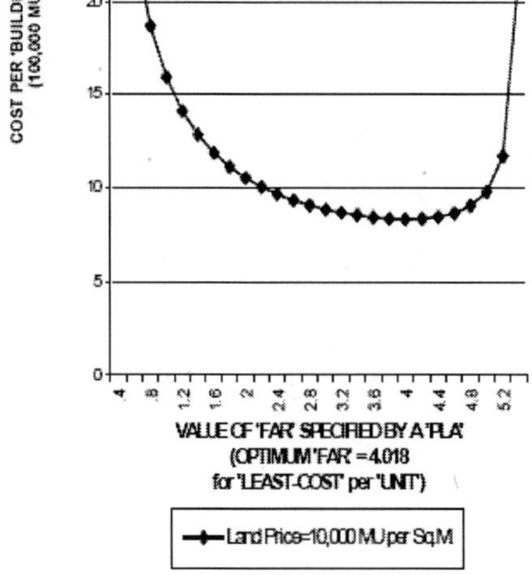

Figure 2. Variation in cost per 'building-unit' with 'FAR' (same built & open space per 'unit').

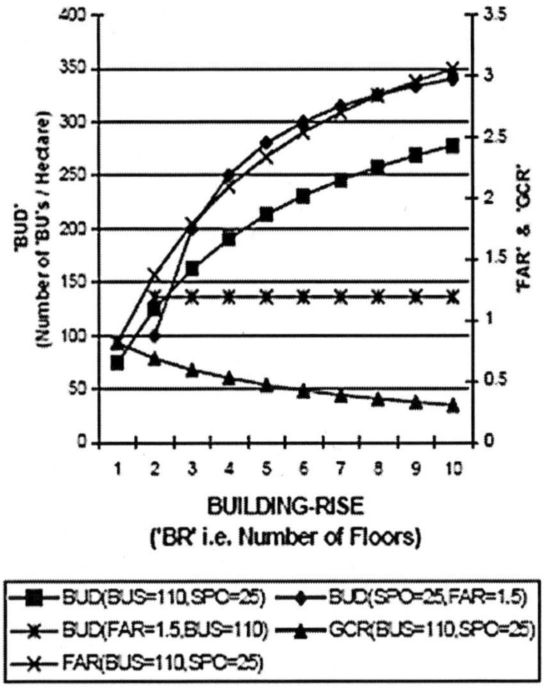

Figure 3. Variation of Density('BUD'),'FAR' & 'GCR' with Building-rise('BR').

Computer graphics allows communication through pictures, charts and diagrams, which are much more meaningful alternatives to the typewriter's string of symbols and alphanumeric expressions. Thus, the information's in the above alphanumeric table containing 16 values of FAR, could be communicated much more meaningfully in a graphic form through a chart or diagram as shown in Figure 2, where all the FAR values between 0.5 and 5.45 are represented giving a much wider picture. Moreover, the diagram clearly indicates that it is an optimisation problem giving the Least Built-Unit-Cost for an unique value of FAR i.e. Optimum FAR, and the user can find this value from the diagram without using the complicated mathematical expression for the same.

Using the above Numeric-Graphic Model a planner-designer can also: (1) determine interaction between the urban 'Built-Form-Elements' (BFE), (2) carry out 'Sensitivity-Analysis', choosing an appropriate set of independent and dependent design variables and the 'Iteration Model', (3) select desired values of 'BFE', using 'Sensitivity-Analysis' in context of '*Urban-Dynamics*', and (4) determine 'Optimal Design' of Urban-Built-Form in a site-specific-case. To carry out such tasks the Software "CAUB/CADUB" incorporates 10 'Iteration Models' depending on the set of design variables chosen, as independent (i.e. user want to input any desired value) or, as dependent (i.e. dependent on the values assigned to independent variables by the user). Using different Iteration Models the Interaction between the Building-Rise (BR) and Built-Unit-Density (BUD) is determined and shown graphically in Figure 3 below, where three possible cases (i.e. adopting constant values of independent variables of: (i) BUS-SPO, (ii) SPO-FAR, and (iii) FAR-BUS, while BR is changed), are shown. Using such results particularly in graphic form, *Planners* and *Designers* can develop an *insight* into the inter-relationships between different urban 'Built-Form-Elements' like BR (BR) and Built-Unit-Density (BUD), including Costs, for *rational decision-making based on scientific relationships,* and thus, avoid the frequent *generalized-prescription* in the *Conventional Planning-Practice* and *Policy* direction regarding Urban-Built-Form, which may be erroneous as discussed later. Each Iteration Model can carry out numerous planning and design analysis covering both *numeric* and *graphic* sessions to find a planning and design solution in graphic form i.e. physical design, fulfilling the given planning-design parameters and standards in numeric terms such as: Built-Space, Open-Space, Built-Unit-Cost and so on, acceptable to all *stakeholders*, including the *User-Citizens* in a site-specific situation.

The Software "CAUB/CADUB", which allows carrying out both Numerical Iteration Session, and after getting Numerical Out-Put Results Loading of the Graphic Program to carry out Drawing Session, is developed to help this process. This is illustrated with one application example presented below.

4.2.2. Urban Planning And Design Analysis Using Numeric-Graphic Model –An Illustrative Example

Software "CAUB/CADUB" incorporates a number of Iteration Models based on the above Numeric-Graphic Model. Application of the Software for Computer Aided Planning and Design Analysis allowing conversion of each Numeric Design into a Graphic Design is illustrated below with an example. An urban user-citizen is generally very much concerned with maximizing Built-Unit-Space (BUS) within a given affordable cost. Hence, such an user may like to analyse a number of potential solutions to determine an acceptable solution within the given affordable cost and fulfilling other desired parameters like open-space, building-rise and so on. Iteration Model-8 in Software "CAUB/CADUB" permits such analysis. Accordingly, Choosing the Iteration Model-8 and entering the desired Input-Values in response to the computer prompt in each cycle of Iteration, a *Numerical Planning Solution* is displayed as output by the Software prompting the user (or all *participating stakeholders*) to indicate the acceptability of the *Numerical Planning Solution* for that cycle. If not acceptable the cycle is repeated entering new input values by the user (s) until an acceptable *Numerical Planning Solution* is displayed and chosen by the user and the Numerical Iteration Session is closed. One such *Numerical Planning Solution* given by the Software is shown below:

SUMMARY OF "CAUB" RESULTS (i.e. *Numerical Solution)* IN THE INSTANT CASE ARE:

ITERATION MODEL CHOSEN (to find BUS for given BUC):	MODEL-8: INTERACTION/ SENSITIVITY (COST+PHY.)
INDEPENDENT DESIGN VARIABLES ('IDV'):	FAR, B.UNIT-COST (BUC), K, BUILDIING-RISE (BR), LAND-PRICE (LP), BASE-PLNTH.AREA RATE (CPAR)
DEPENDENT DESIGN VARIABLES ('DDV'):	BUILT-SPACE (BUS), OPEN-SPACE (SPO), GR.CV.RATIO, AND DENSITY

INPUT PARAMETERS WITH VALUES CHOSEN BY USER:

FAR= 1.50 BUILT-UNIT-COST (BUC)= 800000 MU BUILDING-RISE (BR)= 4
LAND-PRICE (LP)= 5000.0 MU/SQ.M. CPAR= 5000.0 MU/SQ.M. K= 0.0250
ITMODEL= 8 INCHOICE= 10 MU= MONETARY UNITS (i.e. Rupees, Dollars etc.)

OUTPUT PARAMETERS WITH VALUES GIVEN BY THE COMPUTER:

GROSS-PLINTH-AREA-RATE (GPAR)=8833.3 MU/SQ.M.
BUILT-UNIT-SPACE (BUS)= 90.57 SQ.M./BU OPEN-SPACE(SPO)= 37.736 SQ.M./BU
GR.CV.RATIO (GCR) = 0.375 DENSITY (B.UNIT-DENSITY i.e. BUD)= 165.62 BU/HECTARE

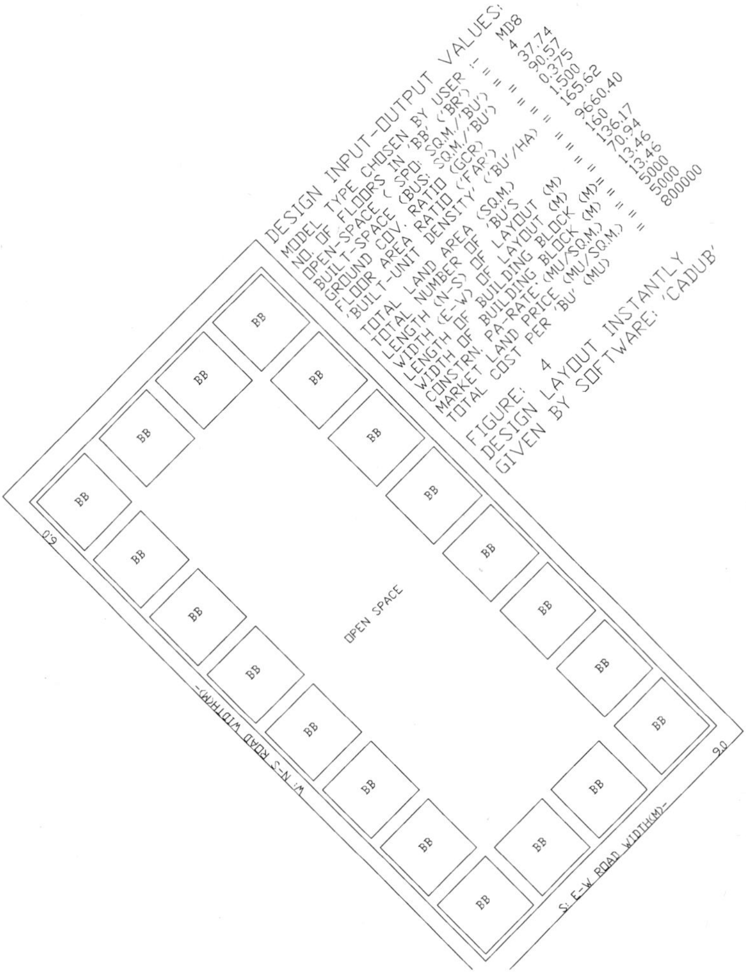

Figure 4. Graphical Design Solution and Numerical Planning Solution.

Accepting the above *Numerical Planning Solution* and closing the Numerical Iteration Session the Graphic Program of the Software is loaded to start the Graphic Iteration Session. Graphic Program prompts the user to put the chosen Model Type, number of dwelling units per floor, number of building blocks (BB) in different direction, and other parameters; when the calculated number of dwelling units and other crucial parameters and dimensions are displayed prompting for acceptance or repeating the Iteration Cycle till these are acceptable to the user. On such acceptance the *Graphical Design Solution* is displayed *instantly*, with or without textual parameters depending on the user choice, for the *Numerical Planning Solution* chosen as above earlier. Figure 4 above shows one such *Graphical Design Solution* exactly matching with the above *Numerical Planning Solution* i.e. Integrating Planning and Design Analysis with Drafting. Thus, modern development of computer technologies including computer graphics allows Planning and Design Analysis of numerous potential solutions to select a particular solution to meet the requirements of *multiple-stakeholders* in a site-specific case.

4.3. Computer-Aided Design by Optimisation and Computer Graphics

The human mind confronting a task or problem can recognize more than one course of action (alternatives) followed by the selection (*decision*) of what is considered the best action, using a measure of effectiveness, often involving a value judgment. Thus, in the above Planning and Design Analysis, a designer can develop one possible solution based on the adopted options, and by repeating this design analysis process using different options and conditions many more possible solutions i.e. alternative solutions can be developed which may appear equally acceptable. However, if a unique optimized design solution were desired relevant *Optimization Techniques* would have to be used, adopting an appropriate measure of effectiveness.

Operations Research (OR), which is often called 'quantitative common sense', is the application of scientific methods to the study of alternatives in a problem situation, with a view to obtaining a quantitative basis for arriving at a best solution [21,22]. This is quite relevant in AEC sector like housing and urban development where architects, engineers and other *urban professionals* and *user-citizens* have to interact to select an alternative from among many alternatives, frequently with different *efficiency-indicators*. Essential characteristics of OR/*Optimization* are its emphasis on *models* (indicating physical depiction of a problem), *goals* (measure of effectiveness), *variables*, *constraints*, and putting them in *mathematical terms* i.e. a *generative system*. Development of *small-scale* models to address a particular Policy problem is often suggested. This is very relevant in urban management, involving building and urban development, requiring both "descriptive" models, if they are designed only to describe the relationships between *variables* in a problem, or "*optimizing*" models designed to lead to selection of best course of action among available alternatives. The author developed earlier a number of descriptive models for shelter design and analysis [18]. In addition to the above Descriptive Numeric-Graphic Model, a number of Optimizing Urban Development Models have also been developed and presented elsewhere [2-10].

Optimization is a *three-step rational decision-making process* i.e. knowledge of the system, finding a measure of system effectiveness and choosing those values of the system variables that yield *optimum* effectiveness. Developing the descriptive model could be the first step of the *Optimization* process i.e. acquiring knowledge of the system. A problem can be *Maximized* for benefit/profit or *Minimized* for cost/loss, and which is desired is a matter of statement. Urban development is both a physical and a socio-economic system and may have conflicting goals/ viewpoints, which need to be resolved using *Optimization* both in qualitative (judged by human preference) and quantitative (using exact mathematical means) terms. Economic *optimization* has to consider human values expressible in quantitative form even if indirectly. For example, the cost difference of given built-space between chosen development types, say between low-rise and medium-rise urban development, could be an indirect measure for qualitative evaluation of these two types of development, while selecting the preferred alternative, with the *participation* of *user-citizen* using collaborative **IT** (Information Technology) -Tools.

Optimization theory is more than a set of numerical recipes for finding optima. By studying various optimization techniques, each suitable for different quantitative situations (even if idealized), one often discerns general *decision rules* appropriate to problems, and can develop an *insight* in recognizing the proper form of an optimal solution even when a problem is not completely formulated in mathematical terms. One advantage of such optimization study is that it can foster recognition of information valuable enough to be gathered to depict a system well enough for it to be optimized (say, bringing agreement on the measure of effectiveness and expressing its quantitative dependence on system variables), thus, help apply *Optimization* in a problem solution. Such an approach is *crucial* to achieve a *resource-efficient* and *equitable* problem solution in the AEC sector (e.g. housing and urban development, urban infrastructure, structural engineering and so on).

Accordingly, a number of such Optimizing Models for Housing and Urban Development Systems are developed and published elsewhere, covering a wide domain of problems in Built-Environment (). These Models give stress on efficient and effective use of resources at urban development project level, to enhance both *Productivity* (i.e. *Efficiency & Effectiveness*) and Social *Responsiveness* to help solve urban problems *Resource-Efficiently*, improving the performance of Urban Organizations in this regard including profitability. *Optimizing Models* are of following two types:

1. Least-Cost Optimizing Models (LCO Models)- this can be used to obtain Least-Cost Design of urban development system, for a given Minimum Acceptable Built-Unit-Space i.e. Built-Space per Built-Unit.
2. Most-Benefit Optimizing Models (MBO Models)- this can be used to obtain Maximum-Built-Unit-Space Design of urban development system, for a given Investment or Affordable Cost Limit. As Sale-Proceeds of a Real Estate are generally proportionate to the Built-Space, that is Maximized by a MBO Model, it can also be called "Maximum Profit Model" for developers and builders in the building and urban sector.

In the above Computer Aided Design Optimisation process Computer Graphics and particularly the Interactive Computer Graphics and Geometric Modelling plays a key role to make it feasible which is extremely difficult in conventional and traditional design methods. Application of such concepts in AEC operations taking housing and urban development (an important area affecting the *quality of life* of people) as examples, is outlined earlier, where urban development modelling for planning analysis and design optimisation are presented, and the salient features of the Application Software: "HudCAD" to carry out such tasks is also described along with a number of illustrative application examples [8,10]. Here, an Optimisation Model taking structural engineering (Reinforced-Concrete Beam Design) as an example is shown below.

4.3.1. Optimization In Structural Engineering-A Model For Least-Cost Design Of Reinforced Concrete Beam

Optimization in structural engineering is of special interest to civil engineers. It is possible to apply the concept of Integrated Computer-Aided-Design by Optimization in structural engineering to attain more productivity. To promote Integrated CAD by Optimization in this area, author has developed a number of such *optimizing models* published elsewhere [5,6]. One of that is presented below.

Minimize the Cost per Unit Length of Beam= $y(x) = c_1 x_1 + c_2 x_2 x_3 + c_3 x_2 + c_4 x_3$

Subject to:

$$a_1 x_1^{-1} x_3 x_5 \leq 1 \qquad (4)$$

(*Constraint* for Equilibrium)

$$a_2 x_4^{-1} + a_3 x_2 x_3 x_4^{-1} \leq 1 \qquad (5)$$

(*Constraint* for bending moment compatibility)

$$a_4 x_2^{-1} x_3^{-1} x_4 x_5^{-1} + a_5 x_2^{-1} x_5 \leq 1 \qquad (6)$$

(*Constraint* for Bending moment)

$$a_6 x_3^{-1} \leq 1 \qquad (7)$$

(*Constraint* for Beam width)

$$x_1, x_2, x_3, x_4, x_5 > 0 \qquad (8)$$

(Non-negativity *constraint*)

c_1, c_2, c_3, c_4, a_1, a_2, a_3, a_4, a_5, and a_6 ;are the model constants related to the cost parameters and the prescribed design conditions. Here, c_1, c_2, c_3, and c_4 are cost-coefficients due to volume of tensile steel reinforcement (MU/cm^3), volume of concrete (MU/cm^3), shuttering along the vertical surfaces of bean (MU/cm^2), and the shuttering along the horizontal surface of bean (MU/cm^2), respectively. Here, a_1 is related to yield strength of tensile steel reinforcement, and compressive strength of concrete; a_2 relates to applied bending moment; a_3 relates to beam span and density of concrete for self-weight bending moment; a_4 relates to the compressive strength of concrete and the capacity reduction factor [12,13]; a_5 defines the centroid of concrete compression; and a_6 defines the minimum acceptable width of beam.

Here, the Model *variables* are:

x_1 = Optimum area of tensile steel reinforcement (cm^2)

x_2 = A variable giving the optimum effective depth of the beam (cm)

x_3 = A variable giving the optimum width of the beam (cm)

x_4 = A variable defining the total applied bending moment including that due to self-weight of beam

x_5 = A variable defining the depth of equivalent rectangular stress block.

Computer Graphics plays a very key role in the development and implementation of such optimization models in terms of geometric modeling of schematic beam design and providing instantly the *graphic outputs* (Drafting/Drawing) after converting the numerical design obtained by solving the above optimization model. The C++ Program Sub-Modules, incorporated in the Software: "RCCAD" for Integrated CAD by Optimization in Structural Engineering, solves, in no time, such *Optimizing Models* for Structural Design *Optimization*, and converts results into *graphic outputs* (Drafting and Drawing), as shown below in illustrative examples.

4.3.2. An 'Application Software' For Integrated Computer Aided Optimal Design And Drafting In Structural Engineering (Reinforced Concrete Beam)

Similar to Application Software: "HudCAD" presented earlier, on loading and typing "RCCAD" in the Text Part of Computer Screen [28,31], the Application Software: "RCCAD", developed for Integrated Computer Aided Optimal Design of RCC Sections, prompts the Designer or User to select a specific Module, with the following message appearing in the Graphic Part of the Computer Screen:

WELCOME TO ::

// RCCAD //

A SOFTWARE FOR "REINFORCED CONCRETE (RC)
COMPUTER-AIDED-DESIGN"TO ACHIEVE LEAST-COST.
"RCCAD",HAS 2 PARTS: (I)"NUMERIC OPTIMIZATION",
AND (II)"GRAPHIC COMPONENT", WHICH CONVERTS
INSTANTLY THE "NUMERIC DESIGN" TO "DRAWING".
SOFTWARE "RCCAD" HAS NUMBER OF MODELS.
SELECT 'NUMERIC' ,OR, 'GRAPHIC' OPTION AND,
A MODEL TO RUN AS PER YOUR REQUIREMENT.

Similar to Application Software: "HudCAD" and "CAUB/CADUB", the Application Software: "RCCAD" for Integrated Computer Aided Optimal Design of RCC Sections can be used for Computer Aided Design Analysis and Optimization allowing conversion of each Numeric Design into a Graphic Design, and thus, help to analyze a number of potential solutions to determine an acceptable solution fulfilling the given design condition(s). Thus, on choosing an appropriate Model and entering the desired Input-Values in response to the computer prompt in each cycle of Iteration, the Software displays a Numerical Design Solution as output and prompts the designer to indicate the acceptability of the Numerical Solution for that cycle. If not acceptable the cycle is repeated entering new input values by the designer until an acceptable *Numerical Solution* is displayed and chosen by the user and the numerical iteration session is closed. Thereafter, the "*graphic iteration session"* or *"drawing session"* is started to convert Numeric Design into a Graphic Design/Drawing and Engineering Drafting.

Adopting the above procedure comparative Graphic Designs and Drawings (i.e. Engineering Drafting of the drawings) of RCC beams given by Software "RCCAD" using:- (1) conventional design method [12,13] and (2) the least-cost *optimal* design method (using *optimizing models* like the one presented above) incorporated in the software is shown in Figure 5. It may be seen that the conventional design is 17.86% costlier than the Least-Cost *Optimal* Design for the same input design conditions, highlighting the benefits of applying Integrated CADD by Optimization in Civil and Structural Engineering practices.

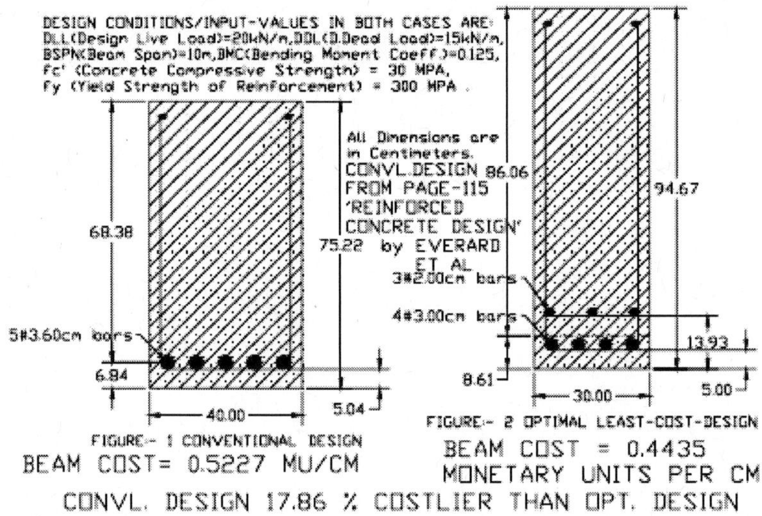

Figure 5. Least-Cost Optimal Design Drawing Of RCC Beam Given By "RCCAD", Showing Specified Input Design Conditions

4.4. Architectural and Engineering Drafting

Drafting is the documentation of the computer aided design process from the initial sketches and conceptual designs in geometric modeling and analysis to the final presentation or working drawings of full-scale architectural and engineering projects. A fully Integrated CAD system should be able to convert all end results of a planning and design process (incorporating design analysis and optimization) into final presentation or working drawings in architectural and engineering projects in AEC sector. However, this will need lot of research and development in the AEC sector. With the ongoing Information Technology revolution and advances made in CAD techniques in different sectors, drafting can be paperless with computer monitors displaying drawings as required, which can be instantly transmitted to the sites and other desired locations through the electronic means. Figure 5 above illustrates engineering drafting using computer graphics. Similarly, Figures-1 & 4 above are architectural and planning drafting, while Figures 6 & 7 below are architectural, engineering and planning drafting.

4.5. Participatory Urban Planning and Design Using Operations Research Tools for More Effective Urban Planning Policies

Application of the concept of Operations Research (OR) in Urban Development Planning and Design Policy Analysis is illustrated in various papers using the "descriptive" and "optimizing models" for urban built-form, housing and urban development, incorporated in the Application Software's "CAUB/CADUB" and "HudCAD", some of which are also presented there [8,9,10]. In section 4.2 Figures 2 & 3 were presented to show the utility of computer graphics for communication through charts and diagrams. Here, the same diagrams, namely, FAR and Built-Unit-Cost Interaction and Building-Rise-Density Interaction are used as two example case studies for urban planning policy analysis, and to show how such tools can be used in participatory urban planning and design. These examples are selected because there are lots of misconceptions with regard to these issues even at the highest *Policy Level* in some countries like India (e.g. National Commission on Urbanization formed by the Government of India). These interactions are analyzed using the above descriptive Numeric-Graphic Operations Research Models, and the above Software's.

4.5.1. FAR & Built-Unit-Cost Interaction- Urban Management And Housing And Urban Development Planning And Design Policy Implications

The above descriptive models could also incorporate easily the unit land-price and building construction costs, to derive the total cost per Built-Unit (i.e. Building-Unit-Cost/ Built-Unit-Cost, or BUC) considering the prevailing market land price, and thus, the effect of a prescribed planning regulation, like FAR, on the BUC could be determined instantly to confirm feasibility/acceptability of such planning regulations with people's (user citizens) participation (bottom-up approach), rather that imposing such regulations from top (usual top-down approach) which may not work. Application results of Module "CAUB"(of Application CAD Software: "CAUB/CADUB"), which incorporates the unit land-price and building construction costs to derive the total cost per Built-Unit and the *scientific-relationships* between built-form-elements, land-price & building construction costs, is shown in Figure 2 above (adopting land price of 10000 Monetary Units (MU) per m^2, BUS=110 m^2, SPO=20 m^2). Figure 2 shows the relationship (*non-linear*) between the 'FAR' and 'Building-Unit Cost', indicating that the respective BU-Costs at FAR of 0.846 (minimum feasible 'FAR' keeping above values of BUS and SPO, unchanged), and 0.5 (frequently specified by a Planning Authority ('PLA'), requiring an increased SPO = 110 m^2, even for a single-storey development), are 2.14 times and 3.2 times the Minimum-BU-Cost occurring *at the Optimum FAR* = 4. 018 (derived by "CAUB"). Such cost variations only due to *Planning Regulations* may be even higher at higher land prices. Urban Planning Authorities (PLA's) in many countries like India continue to keep the *Planning Regulations* unchanged, say since the first Master Plan prepared in 60's (thus, insisting and trying to enforce a low FAR prescribed 50-60 years back) irrespective of the land price increase to astronomical figures since then (even by 1000 times in some cities, and consequent astronomical increase in BU-Cost), creating huge *inefficiency* and *inequity* and the consequent housing and urban problems leading to the Public Interest Litigations (PIL), which in many cases receives attention even at the highest National Judiciary.

Application Results highlights the utility of the Integrated CAD Application Software like above to help better *planning-design-decisions* to achieve *efficiency* and *equity* in building, housing and urban development as part of *Integrated Urban Management. Hence, it is highly desirable that such Urban Planning Development problems are seen as part of Integrated Urban Management Urban Professionals start using Modern Management Techniques like OR/CAD as above to attain a Resource-Efficient and Equitable problem solution.*

4.5.2. Building-Rise-Density Interaction – Urban Management And Building And Urban Development Planning And Design Policy Implications

The variations of Density (i.e. BUD or Built Unit Density), FAR, and GCR with the variation in Building-Rise (i.e. BR) are shown in Figure 3 (produced by "CAUB" using *scientific-relationships* between built-form-elements) below. Figure 3 indicates that in None of the 3 possible cases (i.e. adopting constant values of independent variables of: (i) BUS-SPO, (ii) SPO-FAR, and (iii) FAR-BUS, while BR is changed) a Low-Rise leads to a High-Density. This is *quite contrary to the frequent generalized-prescription* of "*Low Rise High Density (LRHD) Built-Form*" in the *Conventional Planning-Practice* and *Policy* even at the *Highest National Level* [25]! Density can be increased with "Low-Rise" (which also increases the BU-cost creating *inefficiency* due to less sharing of *horizontal-diaphragms*, foundation costs etc., compared to "Medium-Rise"), only by reducing BUS or the SPO (and by increasing the GCR). This may not be acceptable to people and *User-Citizens* who are important *stakeholders* in the urban operations, if they are informed (for an *informed-decision-making* with *transparency*) of such BU-cost increase and BUS-SPO reduction (creating *inequity*), while giving such *pre-conceived prescriptions*. To overcome such limitations of conventional practice to achieve *efficiency* and *equity*, it is imperative for a *Policy* to use Computer-Aided Planning and Design Techniques like Software's "CAUB/CADUB" and "HudCAD" discussed earlier.

The above results show that only due to the Planning-Regulation i.e. FAR specified by a Planning- Authority (entirely within its control) there is very large increase in Cost per BU, even though adequate open space - a basic objective of such Regulations - is achieved even at the Optimum FAR minimizing the Cost/Building-Unit. Such large cost-variations are difficult to be ignored by User-Citizens and other Stakeholders, who would like to maximize "productivity" (output-input ratio) along with the desired environmental standards. This may be one of the reasons for frequent illegal-constructions which may be minimal if User-Citizens are convinced, through Informed-Participation (using Computer Software's such as "CAUB/CADUB" and collaborative Information Technology Tools for Transparency), that the Planning-Regulations do not require any change to achieve their above objectives, including the desired environmental standards.

To secure such *Informed-Participation* of *User-Citizens*, Software "CADUB" cited above can be an useful Tool, as even lay *Citizens* can give *Interactive Inputs* to get both *Numeric* and *Graphic Outputs* for a meaningful participation of such *stakeholders* in the *decision-making* regarding *building-layout-systems* taking into account their *constraints* and *priorities*. But, this is feasible only if a *Policy Decision* exists to include in *professional education* such *Modern Computer-Aided-Planning and Design Techniques* and use it, as part of *Integrated Urban Management*, to overcome the limitations of conventional practice to achieve *Efficiency*, *Effectiveness*, *Equity* and *Optimization* in our Building and Urban Operations. To create such a *capacity*, all Educational Institutions may take a *Policy Decision* to include: "*Computer Aided Planning and Design by Optimization (CAPDO)*" as a full-credit "Course" in the *curricula* of their civil and building engineering, architecture, and urban planning education, and to carry out *Research* to augment the course materials for this subject of study. A suggestive Course Content of this subject of study is at Appendix-A.

4.5.3. Need For Integrated Urban Management Approach And Urban Management Education

An urban area is a highly complex dynamic system of interacting activities and interrelated components involving growth, change and uncertainties requiring application of various management principles, techniques, and tools to manage effectively the interacting activities and interrelated components, recognizing various technological, economic and social issues to promote a *resource-efficient* and *equitable* urban operations and development to improve the *quality of life for all*. One of the distinctive features of an urban area, besides its higher population density and non-agricultural land use, is that its population is characterized by specialization of occupations and of labour with interdependence, requiring extensive managerial organization to provide services deemed essential for civilized survival sustaining productive activities. Urban areas are also subjected to a number of external dynamic influences creating many difficulties and opportunities. Inadequate attention and absence of holistic managerial response to the above interacting factors leads to many urban problems in terms of inadequate access to shelter and urban basic services, proliferation of slums and squatter settlements, inadequate urban infrastructure and transport systems and their high costs, congestion, pollution and other environmental degradations.

As urbanization has many positive impacts outlined above and benefits individuals, communities, businesses, and generates economic wealth of the nation as a whole, going against urbanization may amount to going against the tide of national development and the economic, social, and political forces that spur it. Therefore, efficient urban management is the only way by which urban problems could be minimized while maximizing the above beneficial impacts of urbanization enhancing the role of cities as "engines for economic growth". Governments, Urban Organizations (both in the public and private sector), and Urban Professionals play a key role in the above urbanization process, and a resource-efficient and equitable solution of urban problems and cost-effective urban operations depends very much on the efficiency and effectiveness of the above entities. It is universally recognized that management expertise is very crucial to improve efficiency and effectiveness of any organization to achieve optimal results and goals. Even for the not-for-profit organizations with the goal of public service, management expertise is necessary to accomplish them with minimum of resources or to accomplish as much as possible with a given available resources. However such integrated urban management expertise is very rare in the urban organizations in many countries, which no doubt is one of the crucial factors contributing to the deterioration of urban environment in many countries. Towards this effort a *holistic Course Design* is prepared for "*MBA-Urban Services*", where *Quantitative Methods, OR, and CAD by Optimization* forms an *important* area of *Core Courses* as per National norms [8,9,10]. To create such *capacity* it is *basic* that Universities and other Institutions start such Urban Management Education to produce *Professional Urban Managers*, Urban Organizations decide to employ such *Professional Urban Managers* for more *effective* and *efficient* urban operations, and the *Professional Bodies* take initiatives to remove this *serious gap* in our *Professional Education* related to the Building and Urban Operations creating many urban problems.

4.6. Integrated Computer Aided Design by Optimization

Tedious and voluminous computations involved, in utilizing *Optimization* and Operations Research Techniques and to solve and use *Optimizing Models* discussed above, have prevented their applications in urban development *planning* and *design* in the past. The continued development of cheap and powerful computers with interactive graphics systems has made it possible to perform many planning and design functions integrating graphics with complex computations, design analysis, cost engineering and *Optimization* techniques on a computer. To promote application of such Integrated CAD by *Optimization* in housing and urban development an Application CAD Software named HudCAD, which combines all three elements i.e. *cost,, design optimization and drafting;* solves the above *nonlinear programming models,* and converts *instantly* the *numerical solution* into a *graphic* output, is presented below. The CAD Software permits interactive inputs from the designers, who can obtain *optimal solution* in *numeric/ graphic* form, even if not skilled with such techniques and not computer literate.

Development of "MICROCADD" or "PC-CADD" has revolutionized the fields of design, engineering and drafting because of many advantages over the traditional methods, leading to substantial improvement in productivity [15]. PC-CADD is a more productive approach to design/drafting than manual techniques because of:

1. Faster production of design and data creation
2. Faster data manipulation including graphic data, taking little time in correcting and revising designs and documentation of those designs
3. Faster, more convenient data storage
4. Faster data output including graphic output
5. Instant linkage and conversion of optimal design in numerical terms into a graphic output, thus facilitating application of optimization techniques for resource-efficiency

The area of "Architectural design and drafting-engineering-construction (AEC) " ranks relatively low in PC-CADD systems by application [15]. This is mainly because Integrated CAD in AEC rarely forms part of education curricula in developing countries (e.g. India,) and commercial CAD systems rarely incorporate all components of Integrated CAD to deal with all aspects of design. An Integrated CAD System should have five components: (i) Geometric Modeling, (ii) Cost Engineering, (iii) Design Analysis and Design Optimization, (ivi) Drafting/Drawing, and (v) Data Management, Storage and Transfer. But, most microcomputer-based commercial CAD systems are constructed primarily to perform only geometric modeling and drafting and their performance is effectively limited to what is included in them [19]. CAD primarily depends on: (i) system software - supplied with the hardware, and (ii) application software - available commercially or to be developed in-house. Use of such modern planning, design, and management techniques can increase in AEC only with the development of more and more sophisticated Software's, particularly application software's for Optimal Design, decision support systems and data base management, stressing the use of Information Technology, especially to secure User-Citizen Participation in Planning and Design in urban development. Towards this effort the author is doing research, developed a number of Descriptive and Nonlinear Programming Optimizing Models for

Building/Housing/Urban Development and also for Structural Engineering, published elsewhere. Now Application Software: HudCAD (in Modular form) is being developing, linking these Descriptive and Universal Optimizing Models, as an Integrated Computer Aided Planning & Design System (giving stress on Design Optimization), to help adopt an Integrated Urban Management Approach to improve Efficiency, Equity & Social Responsiveness in the Housing and Urban Development Operations [9,10]. The salient feature of Application Software: HudCAD (Housing and Urban Development Computer Aided Design) for Integrated Computer Aided Design by Optimization, is outlined below detailing its utility as an IT-TOOL to achieve Efficiency, Equity and Social Responsiveness in housing & urban development process with Participation of Multiple Stakeholders. Similarly, Integrated CAD Application Software for Structural Design Optimization is also being developed. Using one Software Module, incorporating "optimizing model" for Least-Cost Design of Reinforced Concrete Beam presented above, application of concept of Integrated Computer-Aided-Design by Optimization in structural engineering is also illustrated above i.e. Figure 5.

As outlined above, CAD has many components, and the principles and mathematical formulations of computer graphics, geometric modeling, interactive graphics, architectural and engineering drafting, design analysis, and design optimizations are essential elements of a modern CAD system for any sector including the AEC sector. Similarly, cost engineering would be an important component of a CAD system where cost is a consideration for design, as in the AEC sector, in which cost is paramount in many cases to attain a *resource-efficient* and effective problem solution. Data management, storage and transfer should also form part of a CAD system, to permit efficient data management for speedy information handling and decision-making resulting to higher productivity (i.e. efficiency and effectiveness), which is one of the basic objectives of CAD. As earlier mentioned Planning and Design needs to be viewed as a *problem solving process* in a resource-efficient manner. This view is especially relevant in Architecture, Planning, and Civil Engineering (say, Building/ Housing/ Urban Services) i.e. AEC sector, consuming huge *Resources* and affecting the *quality of life* of people in many countries. In view of above, all the components of CAD needs to be integrated in the form of a comprehensive planning and design tool i.e. as an Integrated CAD System and applied in a specific problem situations to maximize the benefits of CAD in solving a problem in a resource-efficient and effective manner.

Ideally, an Integrated CAD system should cover the entire portion of the professional planning and design practices in different sectors. To build such a comprehensive tool suitable for specific design needs and for a specific sector, a lot of research and development is necessary, consuming lot of time and money. There are many commercial CAD software packages named as turnkey systems for some sectors, developed by integrating some major components of CAD such as: geometric modeling, design analysis, engineering drafting, and data management, storage, and transfer; but these are very costly. These are created as "black boxes", for practical application requiring no further in-house development or system modification by the user in most cases. Turnkey natures of these systems make it possible to effectively use the systems by the users, having little knowledge or specialized training in software programming. However, many such systems are so costly that they are beyond the reach of most small sized industries, offices, professional organizations or individual professionals. In view of above, there is need for research and development to develop Integrated CAD software's for AEC sector which should be less costly ensuring liberal availability of research results to all concerned including users of Integrated CAD for further development to meet their specific needs as they arise while using such systems by the user.

As building a comprehensive Integrated CAD tool covering all components is an uphill task and very costly, author feels that initially it should include major components such as: (i) geometric modeling, (ii) cost engineering, (iii) planning and design analysis, (iv) design optimization, (v) architectural and engineering drafting/drawing, and (vi) data management, storage, and transfer. Software "HudCAD" is being developed with different Modules covering building design, area planning (Software Modules "CADUB"/ "CAUB"), cost engineering, and so on, incorporating both descriptive and optimizing models for different types of Building/Urban Development. Several Modules of the Software are developed. Each Module for *Integrated Computer Aided Design* has two parts: (i) Numeric, and (ii) Graphic, and carry out all Five major functions of an *Integrated Computer-Aided Design System*, mentioned above. Geometric modeling, which defines an object in terms of geometric properties and arrangement of spaces, is done by including *dimensionless* building-unit/built-unit patterns in different groups in the Graphic Part of the Software. The *Design Analysis* and *Design Optimization* components include both Descriptive and Optimizing Models, and are included in the Numeric Part which also store/transfer data of interest creating data files.

The Numeric Parts are developed as independent Software's in user-friendly C++ language, which solves the Non-linear Programming Optimizing Models (both Least-Cost and Most-Benefit Optimizing Models presented above), Descriptive Models (presented above), and Cost Engineering Models [20]. It generates descriptive/optimal solutions in *alphanumeric* form, complying with the specified *objective* (such as Least-Cost or Most-Benefit Design) and *constraints*, linking various building/ urban planning parameters such as: Built-Space, Density, Open Space, Floor Area Ratio, Ground Coverage Ratio and Cost Engineering (including Construction Specifications, Elemental Costs). It runs cost-engineering program to derive site-specific cost-coefficients, and process the input data for calibrating the *Optimizing Models* by deriving Model Constants for a site-specific case. Cost Engineering Program also carries out data management, storage and transfer functions related to costs. Drafting/ drawing is carried out by a Graphic Program, which uses LISP (AutoLISP) Language for graphic operations. As drawing is the most important medium of building/ housing/ urban planning and design, any *numeric design solution* needs to be converted *Instantly* into drawings to be meaningful to all *stakeholders* and even to lay User Citizens. The Graphic Program carries out this task, and can call Numeric C++ Program when required to generate an acceptable numeric solution before converting it into a graphic solution. Graphic Program also generates/ store/transfer data of interest in the output drawing (presently line drawings). Thus, the Software "HudCAD" covers all five components of an Integrated Computer Aided Design System including Optimization. Typical Least-Cost Optimal Built-Unit Design-Drawing given by "HudCAD", based on integrating all the five components of Integrated CAD cited above, is shown below in Figure 6.

The architectural and engineering drafting of Least-Cost optimal design of BU given by Software "HudCAD" as above is obtained by solving the relevent optimisation model using C++ programming language. The optimisation model solution is based on solution of cost engineering model incorporating site-specific labour and material cost input data, and the Least-Cost i.e. minimum possible cost per BU stated in the above drawing is supported by detailed estimate also generated by the Software instantly.

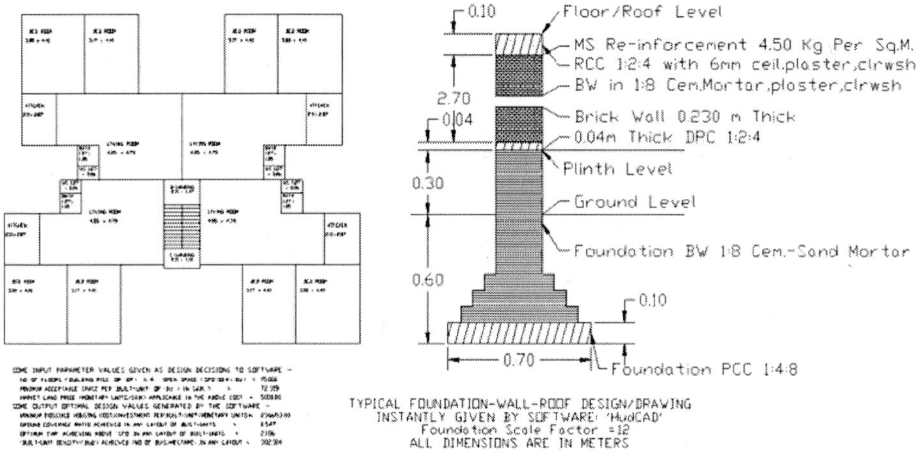

Figure 6. Typical Least-Cost Optimal Built-Unit Design-Drawing Given by “HudCAD”, Integrating all five Components of Integrated CAD.

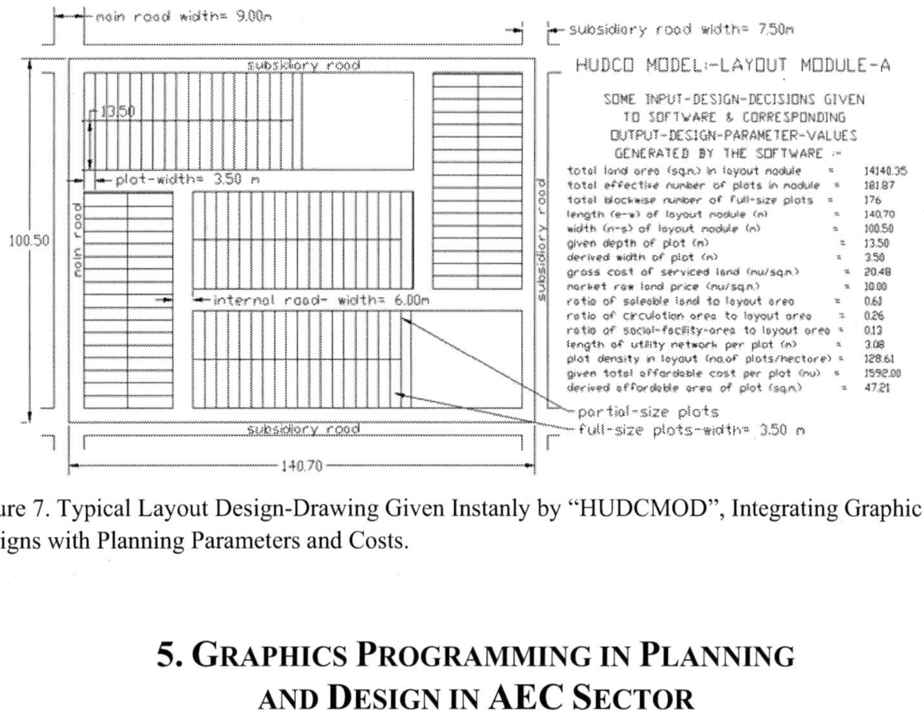

Figure 7. Typical Layout Design-Drawing Given Instanly by “HUDCMOD”, Integrating Graphic Designs with Planning Parameters and Costs.

5. Graphics Programming in Planning and Design in AEC Sector

As mentioned above an Integrated CAD System have five components i.e. (i) Geometric Modeling, (ii) Cost Engineering, (iii) Design Analysis and *Design Optimization*, (iv) Drafting/Drawing, and (v) Data Management, Storage and Transfer. All these components need to be integrated if the system is to be used effectively and efficiently. Design Analysis, *Design Optimization*, and Data Management, Storage and Transfer (to a large extent) would require a high level programming language like C, C++ or FORTRAN for carrying out such tasks and their integration. A graphics system is a collection of hardware and software designed to make it easier to use graphic input and output in computer programs [26]. Graphics software is required to generate graphical images such as Geometric Modeling and Drafting/Drawing. Generally there are two types of graphics software’s, namely, general programming packages and the special purpose application packages [11,33,34]. Extensive set of graphics functions, which are provided by a general programming package, can be used in a high-level programming language like C, C++, and FORTRAN. Thus, using such a general programming package along with a generally accepted standard for computer graphics (such as the Graphical Kernel System or GKS with suitable language binding), would not only permit integration of all the five components in an Integrated CAD package but also enhance its portability. But, this would require lot of research and development that is rare in AEC sector. It is desirable to carry out research in AEC sector to develop such Universal Integrated CAD packages incorporating Optimisation and the accepted standard for computer graphics enhancing portability, and further development and use by various users in diverse hardware systems and in different implementations and applications.

The other type of graphics software is the special purpose application packages such as AutoCAD, which is widely used in AEC sector. Although, using such a graphic software system both the tasks of Geometric Modeling and Drafting/Drawing can be carried out, but the problem of integrating these tasks with the Design Analysis, *Design Optimization*, and Data Management, Storage and Transfer have to be addressed using a suitable graphics programming language or a high level computer programming language as above. Fortunately, AutoCAD supports AutoLISP, which is implementation of the LISP programming language. Using AutoLISP in combination with a high-level computer programming language like C++, it is possible to integrate Geometric Modeling and Drafting/Drawing tasks with the Design Analysis, *Design Optimization*, and Data Management, Storage and Transfer. This approach has been adopted in developing the Integrated CAD Application Software: "HudCAD", mentioned above. However, simple Planning and Design Analysis using OR Models in terms of simple algebraic expressions, and the corresponding Drafting/Drawing can be integrated using only AutoLISP. This is illustrated below with an example AutoLISP CAD Application Software: "HUDCMOD".

5.1. Application of Graphics Programming Using Autolisp - An Example

As mentioned above essential characteristics of OR/*Optimization* are its emphasis on *models* indicating physical depiction of a problem and describing the relationships between *goals*, *variables*, and *constraints* in *mathematical terms*. Many authors have attempted modeling the urban system and a number of *large-scale* urban models are available in the literature [14, 23]. Development of *small-scale* models to address a particular Policy problem is often suggested. This is very relevant in urban management, involving building and urban development, requiring both "descriptive" and "optimizing" models. Moreover, the relationships between many design-variables connected to cost are often nonlinear, time dependent and physical design related. Hence, it is desirable to develop *small-scale* urban development *models*, linked with physical design and adopting a shorter planning horizon, to permit Planning and Design Analysis with more realistic costs.

To help this process application of the concept of OR in Urban Development Planning and Design Policy analysis is illustrated above using a "descriptive" model developed for Urban Built-Form. Similarly, the author developed earlier a number of descriptive models in terms of simple algebraic expressions for shelter design and analysis [18]. Any large-scale urban layout generally has some basic modules or planning modules, which are repeated to form the whole layout. Hence, by suitable control of the quantitative planning and design efficiency indicators (such as: saleable land ratio, circulation space ratio, open space ratio, social facility space ratio, plot density, quantity and cost of utility networks, cost per unit of saleable land, cost per plot and so on) of such planning modules the character, land use and cost structure of the whole layout can be controlled. Thus, the planning modules must be efficient in terms of saleable land and circulation space to ensure that the layout as a whole is also efficient in terms of these parameters. Similarly, a layout module needs to be designed in physical terms to ensure that the cost of residential plots are affordable by intended users (say urban poor) which can be ensured if the given affordable cost is taken as independent design variable in the design of a layout module to give the plot size within the above affordable cost, and selecting suitable mix of other planning and design parameter values (such as open space per plot, utility network specification and so on) in a number of iterations, and thus, carry out a *planning and design analysis* before deciding the physical design of the layout module. Descriptive models in terms of simple algebraic expressions given in HUDCO MODEL were intended to permit such *planning and design analysis*, which could be only in numeric terms since these models did not have any graphics programming features to make it more meaningful. By Graphics Programming using AutoLISP it is possible to integrate the algebraic expressions with Drafting and Drawing to permit *Planning and Design Analysis* both in *numeric* and *graphic* terms, and obtain cost-effective Layout Planning and Dwelling Designs in terms of physical designs, fulfilling the given cost parameters and environmental standards acceptable to different users and *stakeholders* as per their requirements and priority.

Hudco Model contains a Typology of Planning Modules and Dwelling Options covering a number of Modules and Options, based on a large number of executed projects. Application of Graphics Programming using AutoLISP is illustrated taking the Layout Planning Module-A, one of the many Layout Modules included in the HUDCO MODEL [18]. The complete listing of this Graphics Programme i.e. CAD Application Software: "HUDCMOD" using AutoLISP is given in Appendix-B, which can be run by any user who can modify it as per specific requirement, and also, attempt such graphic programming for all Layout Modules and Dwelling Option incorporated in the HUDCO MODEL. Typical layout design drawing given instantly by "HUDCMOD", integrating graphic designs with planning parameters and costs is shown in Figure 7 above, where some Input- Design-Decisions given to the Software by a Stakeholder/User/Planner/Designer and the corresponding Output-Design-Parameter Values instantly generated by the Software are also displayed.

6. Conclusion

In recent years, there is tremendous increase in capabilities of computer hardware's and graphics resulting to unparalleled transformations in computers in terms of their capacity to capture data, to analyse, manipulate and store them, to disseminate and communicate information's, and to apply these capabilities in different areas and fields of specialization. Such transformations are occurring with increasing rapidity and frequency in many areas and the rate at which Information Technology (IT) and Computer Applications are spreading to various sectors is extraordinary and has few parallels in technological history. The pervasiveness and cheapness of IT is influencing the way we live, work and enjoys ourselves. Today, information technology and computer application is everywhere shrinking the effects of time and distance and altering the very nature of work in an organization making many writers to view it as the second Industrial Revolution.

As mentioned above Computer Aided Design (CAD) is a vital application area of this ongoing all-pervasive Information Technology Revolution shrinking the effects of time and distance, and altering the very nature of work in an organization. Modern computers can generate and process information on a scope never before possible, and if such information, generated only in alphanumeric form in hundreds of pages it may be of no worth to a human user unable to comprehend them. But these may be very meaningful and extremely useful if presented graphically. Moreover, Computer Graphics is of great help to make computers extremely 'user-friendly' from the outset where computer can be accessed directly in 'user' language, permitting even lay public users without any computer literacy to use it effectively and meaningfully making it feasible to adopt a participatory planning and design to address various social issues. All these are accelerating application of CAD in various fields with recent advances in microcomputer technology, steady decline in cost of computers, and tremendous increase in their computing power and graphic capabilities.

This is equally applicable in Architecture (including Planning), Civil-Building Engineering, and Construction i.e. A-E-C field [11,15,24,29]. As a result of recent advances in microcomputer technology, Engineers, Architects, Planners and Urban Managers everywhere have now access to better and cheaper computer hardware and software to produce sophisticated computer analysis, optimization, graphics and drafting. As a result of tremendous increase in the capabilities of computer hardware and graphics in various fields Computers can play a significant role in addressing various social, environmental and development issues for a just society with informed public participation in the decision-making process on such issues, which is very relevant in AEC, and in this process Computer Graphics can be of great help to make computers extremely 'user-friendly' from the outset where computer is accessed directly in 'user' language, permitting even lay public users without any computer literacy to participate in the decision-making process. This is illustrated with a number of examples presented above indicating the intimate relationships between CAD and Computer Graphics.

Real utility of Computer Aided Design (CAD) and Computer Graphics is no longer confined to just producing sophisticated solid geometry's and more attractive drawing packages only, but can cover many other aspects of design work including optimization to improve productivity and derive other benefits at various operation levels. In this context *Planning and Design* in AEC i.e. Civil Engineering/Buildings/Urban Services need to be viewed as a *problem solving process* forming *Part* (i.e. *Planning Function*) of *Integrated Urban Management* to achieve the *Goal* of *Resource-Efficient* and *Equitable* solution of our mounting urban problems, *Maximizing* the beneficial impacts of urbanization. In this *problem solving process*, which involves *search* through *numerous* potential solutions (*with very large variations in the Resource-Efficiency-Indicators of even 2-3 times* as shown in example problems presented above) to select a particular solution that meets a specified *criteria* or *goal* (e.g. *efficiency & equity*), *Computing* is indispensable. Since, *Operations Research/ Optimization & Computer-Aided Design* are *Basic Techniques* to improve *Efficiency & Effectiveness* [21, 22], it is *Basic* that the Building/ *Urban Professionals* use such *Techniques* to *Discharge* their *Ethical Responsibility/ACCOUNTABILITY* to the *Society or People* to achieve *Efficiency, Effectiveness & Equity* in the use of *huge Resources* (although, inadequate compared to the need with many *claimants*) *committed* by them in their *planning and designs decisions*, to produce building/urban services, and thus, help achieve the above *Goal*.

However, *Optimization*, using such *modern technology*, is rarely applied in our Civil Engineering, Building, Urban Operations, creating many *inefficiencies and inequities* and the consequent urban problems, although, *even the ancients applied Optimization* when population was much fewer, *resource-constraints* much less severe, and *technology* was almost nonexistent. To correct this situation it is suggested that all Educational Institutions may include: "*Computer Aided Planning and Design by Optimization (CAPDO)*" as a full-credit *Course* in the *curricula* of their civil/building engineering, urban planning, architecture education, and to carry out *Research* in this *area* to widen the scope of application of such modern techniques in our building/urban operations in this *new millennium*. This will *EQUIP* students (future building/urban professionals) to *apply* such *modern techniques*, and to adopt an *integrated problem solving approach* in our building/ urban operations to improve the *quality of life for all*, in a *resource-efficient & equitable* manner, in the context of *urban dynamics,* and the *affordability and resource-constraints* at various levels.

REFERENCES

[1] Beightler, C. S., Phillips, D. T. & Wilde, D. J. (1979). "*Foundations of Optimization*", Prentice-Hall, Englewood Cliffs, NJ.

[2] Chakrabarty, B. K. (1988). "A Model for Optimal Design of Dwelling-Layout Systems", Building *and Environment*, Elsevier Science, *vol-23*, no-1.

[3] Chakrabarty, B. K. (1990). "Models for the Optimal Design of Housing Development Systems", *Environment and Planning B: Planning and Design*, Pion, *vol-17*, no-3.

[4] Chakrabarty, B. K. (1991). "Optimization in Residential Land Subdivisions", *Journal of Urban Planning and Development, American Society of Civil Engineers*, *vol-117*, no-1.

[5] Chakrabarty, B. K. (1992). "Models for Optimal Design of Reinforced Concrete Beams", *Computers & Structures*, Pergamon Press, *vol-42*, no-3.

[6] Chakrabarty, B. K. (1992). "A Model for Optimal Design of Reinforced Concrete Beam", *Journal of Structural Engineering*, *American Society of Civil Engineers*, *vol-118*, no-11.

[7] Chakrabarty, B. K. (1996). "Optimal Design of Multifamily Dwelling Development Systems", *Building and Environment*, Elsevier Science, *vol-31*, no-1.

[8] Chakrabarty, B. K. (1998). "Urban management and optimizing urban development models", *Habitat International*, *Elsevier Science*, *vol-22*, no-4.

[9] Chakrabarty, B. K. (2001). "Urban Management: concepts, principles, techniques and education", *Cities*, *Elsevier Science*, *vol-18*, no-5\.

[10] Chakrabarty, B. K. (2007). "Computer-Aided Design in Urban Development and Management-A Software for Integrated Planning and Design by Optimization", *Building and Environment*, Elsevier Ltd, *vol-42*.

[11] Donald Hearn, M. Pauline Baker, (1997). *"Computer Graphics C Version", Pearson Education Inc.*,

[12] Everard, N. J., Tanner, III J. L. (1987). "*Theory and Problems of Reinforced Concrete*

Design", McGraw-Hill, New York.
[13] Fintel, M. (1987). "*Hand Book of Concrete Engineering*", CBS Publishers, Delhi.
[14] Foot, D. (1981). "*Operational Urban Models -An Introduction*", Methuen, New York.
[15] Goetch David, L. (1990). "MicroCADD: Computer-Aided Design and Drafting on Microcomputers", *Prentice-Hall of India*, New Delhi.
[16] Harvey, J. (1987). "*Urban Land Economics*", Macmillan Education Ltd., London.
[17] Hoch, I. (1969). "The three-dimensional city: contained urban space" in "The Quality of Built-environment" S. P. Harvey, (Ed), *Resources for The Future Inc.* Washington DC.
[18] HUDCO, (1982). "*Computer Based Design and Analysis of Affordable Shelter - Hudco Model*", New Delhi.
[19] Hsu, T. & Sinha, D. K. (1992). "Computer -Aided Design: *An Integrated Approach*", West Publishing Company, St.Paul.
[20] Jelen, F. C. & Black, J. H. (1983). "*Cost and Optimization Engineering*", McGraw-Hill Book Company, New York.
[21] Koontz, H. & O'Donnel, C. (1976). "*Management- A System and Contingency Analysis of Managerial Functions*", McGraw-Hill Publishing Company, New York.
[22] Koontz, H. & Weihrich, H. (1990). "*Essentials of Management*", McGraw-Hill Publishing Company, New York.
[23] McLoughlin, J. B. (1969). "*Urban and Regional Planning - A Systems Approach*", Faber and Faber, London.
[24] Mitchell, W. J. (1977). "*Computer-Aided Architectural Design*", Petrocelli/Charter, New York
[25] NCU, (1988). "*Report of The National Commission on Urbanisation*", Volume-II, Government of India Press, New Delhi.
[26] Newman William, M. & Sproull Robert, F (1981). "*Principles of Interactive Computer Graphics*", McGraw-Hill International Book Company, New Delhi.
[27] Nigel Piercy, (1984). "*Management and New Information Technology*" in "The Management Implications of New Information Technology" Nigel Piercy (Ed), Croom Helm, London.
[28] Oliver, W. M. (1990). "*Illustrated AUTOLISP*", BPB Publications, New Delhi.
[29] Ryan, Daniel, L. (1994). "*Computer-Aided Graphics and Design*", Mercel Dekker Inc., New York.
[30] Sanoff Henry, "Integrating Programming (1992), *Evaluation and Participation in Design*", Avebury, Sydney.
[31] Schaefer, A. T. & Brittain, J. L. (1989). "The AutoCAD Productivity Book", *Indian Reprint Edition*, Golgotia Publishers, New Delhi.
[32] Smith, W. F. (1975). "*Urban Development-The Process and The Problems*", University of California Press, Berkeley.
[33] Stevens Roger, T. (1993). "*Graphics Programming in C*", BPB Publications, New Delhi.
[34] Steven Harrington, (1987). "*Computer Graphics - A Programming Approach*", ", McGraw-Hill Publishing Company, New York.

APPENDIX-A

Subject: Computer-Aided Planning and Design by Optimization

A Suggestive Course-Content:

An Overview of Computer-Aided Planning and Design
CAD and Traditional Design
Computerizing the Planning & Design Process
Commercial CAD Systems
Components of Integrated CAD System
Numerical Techniques for CAD
Elements of Computer Graphics & Architectural/Engineering Drafting
Elements of Cost Engineering
Planning and Design Databases
Elements of *Operations Research* (OR) & *Optimization* Techniques
Applications in Planning, Architecture, Building/ Civil Engineering
Planning/Design *Analysis* and *Optimization*
Towards a Theory of *Optimal* Urban Built-Form
Software for Analysis and *Optimization* of Building/Development Control-
Role of Information Technology (IT) for *Citizen Participation*
Managing the *Dynamics* of Urbanization - Applying the
Urban Management *Principles of Flexibility* with Participatory & Collaborative IT-Tools
Models and Computer-Aided Layout Design by *Optimization*
Models and Computer-Aided Building Design by *Optimization*
Models and Computer-Aided Dwelling-Layout System Design by *Optimization*
Models and Computer-Aided Structural Design by *Optimization* - Reinforced Concrete Sections
Computer-Aided Infrastructure Design by *Optimization*
Integrated CADD by *Optimization* from AutoLISP
Interfacing Numeric *Analysis/Optimal* Design & Graphic Design using C++, AutoCAD & AutoLISP;
Automating *Descriptive/Optimal* Design Drawings, Costing & Bill of Materials
Integrative, Multidisciplinary & **Participatory Optimal Planning & Design** with User Interface using IT
Concept of general Graphics Standards to enhance portability of computer graphics programming

APPENDIX-B

; HUDCMOD.LSP

```
; Layout Module Design Generating Program Using Layout-Module:-A in ; HUDCO-Model-1982.
; Developed as a Self-Contained Tool for Analysis & Design of Layout-;Module:-A, Considering ;Various Planning and Design Parameters including ;Costs.
; Developed by Dr. B.K.Chakrabarty
(defun lis2 ()
  (setq i 6.0 su 7.5 m 9.0 o 10.0 r 1.4 d 13.5)
  (princ "\npre-set physical parameters are:i=6.0,su=7.5,m=9.0,o=10.0,r=1.4,d=13.5 ")
 (setq cpp ( strcase (getstring "\ndo you want to change the above values(y/n) ? " )))
 (if (= cpp  "y" )
(progn
 (setq i (getreal "\nenter desired width of internal road(changed)  : " ))
 (setq su (getreal "\nenter desired width of subsidiary road(changed)  : " ))
 (setq m  (getreal "\nenter desired width of main road (changed)  : " ))
 (setq o (getreal "\nenter desired open-space(sfs) per plot(changed): " ))
 (setq r (getreal "\nenter desired layout-module ratio (changed): " ))
 (setq d (getreal "\nenter desired depth of plot (changed): " ))
 (princ "" )
 (setq ci 231.0 cs 281.0 cm 414.0 cl 10.0 pc 1592.0)
 (princ "\npre-set cost parameters are:ci=231.0,cs=281.0,cm=414.0,cl=10.0,pc=1592.0 ")
 (setq ccp ( strcase (getstring "\ndo you want to change the above values(y/n) ? " )))
 (if (= ccp  "y" )
 (progn
 (setq ci (getreal "\nenter desired cost of internal road(changed)  : " ))
 (setq cs (getreal "\nenter desired cost of subsidiary road(changed)  : " ))
 (setq cm  (getreal "\nenter desired cost of main road (changed)  : " ))
 (setq cl (getreal "\nenter desired cost of raw land (changed): " ))
 (setq pc (getreal "\nenter desired affordable cost of plot (changed): " ))
 )
 (princ "" )
 )
 )
 (defun lpar ()
 (setq b (+ (* 6 d) (* 2 i)  su ) )
 (setq l (* b r ) )
 (setq a (* b l ) )
 (setq x (- (* 6 l) ( + (* 4 i) (* 3 su) (* 3 m )  ) ) )
 (setq q2 (+ (* (+ (* 0.5 b) l ) cs ) (* (* 0.5 b) cm ) ( * a cl) ) )
 (setq q1 (* (- (+ (* 2 l) (* 4 d) ) m su ) ci ) )
 (setq q (+ q1 q2) )
 (setq pa (- (/ (* pc x d) q ) o ) )
 (prompt "\naffordable plot size (sq.m.) =  " )
 (princ (eval pa) )
 (getstring "\nput any character to continue : " )
 (setq n (/ (* d x ) (+ pa o) ) )
 (princ (eval n) )
 (setq rn (fix n) )
```

```
(prompt "\nrounded number of total plots in module = " )
(princ (eval rn) )
(getstring "\nput any character to continue : " )
(setq ow (/ o d) )
(setq nplw (/ pa d) )
(setq gplw (+ ow nplw) )
(setq vl (+ (* 4 d) i )  )
(setq hml (- l (+ (* 4 d ) (* 2 i ) (* 0.5 (+ m su) )  )  )  )
(setq hl1 (+ i (* 2 d) ) )
(setq hl2 (+ (* 0.5 m) (* 0.5 su) hl1 ) )
(setq hl (- l  hl2 )  )
(setq tosp (* n o ) )
(setq on 0.5 os 0.5 om 0.001 oe 0.001 owp 0.001)
(princ "\npre-set open space proportions are:on=0.5,os=0.5,om=0.001,oe=0.o01,owp=0.001")
(setq cosp ( strcase (getstring "\ndo you want to change the above values(y/n) ? " )))
(if (= cosp  "y" )
(progn
(prompt "\nput desired open space proportions(0.001 if 0)each block(total all blocks=1) " )
(setq on (getreal "\nput desired open space proportion-north e-w block(on-changed):" ))
(setq os (getreal "\nput desired open space proportion-south e-w block(os-changed):" ))
(setq om (getreal "\nput desired open space proportion-middle e-w block(om-changed):" ))
(setq oe (getreal "\nput desired open space proportion-east n-s block(oe-changed):" ))
(setq owp (getreal "\nput desired open space proportion-west n-s block(owp-changed):" ))
)
(princ "" )
)
(setq onl (/ (* tosp on) (* 2 d)  ) )
(setq osl (/ (* tosp os) (* 2 d)  ) )
(setq oml (/ (* tosp om) (* 2 d)  ) )
(setq oel (/ (* tosp oe) (* 2 d)  ) )
(setq owl (/ (* tosp owp) (* 2 d)  ) )
(if (< hml oml )
(progn
(setq omlo oml)
(setq oml hml)
(setq owl (+ owl (- omlo hml) ) )
)
(princ "" )
)
(setq npln (/ (- hl onl) nplw  ) )
(setq rnpn (fix npln) )
(setq npls (/ (- hl osl) nplw  ) )
(setq rnps (fix npls) )
(setq nplm (/ (- hml oml) nplw  ) )
(setq rnpm (fix nplm) )
(setq nple (/ (- vl oel) nplw  ) )
(setq rnpe (fix nple) )
(setq npw (/ (- vl owl) nplw  ) )
```

```
(setq rnpw (fix npw) )
 )
(defun dimen ()
(setq ds 15.0)
(prompt "\npre-set dimension scale is = " )
(princ (eval ds) )
(setq cds (strcase (getstring "\ndo you want to change dimension scale ? (y/n): " )))
( if (= cds "y")
(setq ds (getreal "\nenter desired dimension scale (changed)  : " ))
(princ   "" )
)
(command "dim" "dimscale" ds  )
(command)
(dim)
(command)
 )
(defun dim()
(setq w1 (list (car ip) (- (cadr ip) 12.0 ) ) )
(setq v1 (list (- (car ip) 12.0 ) (cadr ip ) ) )
(command "dim" "hor" ip f0 w1 sllyt )
(command "dim" "ver" v1 f1 v1 swlyt )
(setq pp1 (list (+ (car ps3) 0.25) (- (cadr ps3) 2) ) )
(setq d1 (list (car d) (- (cadr d) 5.5 ) ) )
(setq d2 (list (+ (car d1) 2.0) (cadr d1) ) )
(setq pp2 (list (- (car ps4) 2 ) (+ (cadr ps4) 4) ) )
(setq d3 (list (car d1) (- (cadr d1) 5 ) ) )
(setq d4 (list (+ (car d3) 2.0) (cadr d3) ) )
(setq dimm1 (list (car cornn) (+ (cadr cornn) 4 ) ) )
(setq dimm2 (list (car dmm2 ) (+ (cadr dmm2) 4 ) ) )
(setq dims1 (list (car crne) (+ (cadr crne) 4 ) ) )
(setq dims2 (list (car dms2) (+ (cadr dms2) 4 ) ) )
(setq mn1 (list (+ (car dimm1) 2.5) (+ (cadr dimm1) 4) ) )
(setq mn2 (list (+ (car dimm1) 1.0) (cadr mn1) ) )
(setq mrwtxt (strcat "main road width= " sm "m" ) )
(setq srwtxt (strcat "subsidiary road width= " ss "m " ) )
(setq irwtxt (strcat "internal road- width= " si "m " ) )
(setq pptxt (strcat "partial-size plots" ) )
(setq fptxt (strcat "full-size plots-width= " splw " m ") )
(setq inr1 (list (car ps0) (+ (cadr ps0) (* 0.5 i) ) ) )
(setq inr2 (polar inr1 pi i) )
(command "dim" "hor" dmm2 cornn mn1 mrwtxt )
(command "dim" "hor" dims1 dims2 dims2 srwtxt )
(command "dim" "hor" inr2 inr1 inr1 irwtxt )
(command "dim" "leader" pp1 d1 d2  ""  pptxt )
(command "dim" "leader" pp2 d3 d4  ""  fptxt )
(setq pwtxt (strcat "plot-width= " splw " m ") )
(setq pwtp (polar plm1 (* 0.5 pi) (* 0.5 i) ) )
(command "dim" "hor" pl3 pl4 pwtp pwtxt )
```

```
 (command "dim" "ver" pl1 pl2 pl2 spld )
 (command)
 )
(defun plot ()
 (command "zoom" "a" )
 (setq tewpl (* (+ rnpn rnps rnpm ) 2 ) )
 (setq tnspl (* (+ rnpe rnpw ) 2 ) )
 (setq tnpl (+ tnspl tewpl) )
 (prompt "\nrounded number(integer value) of total-plots (all blocks)= " )
 (princ (eval tnpl) )
 (getstring "\nput any character to continue 1 : " )
 (setq dx nplw dy d )
 (setq num rnpn)
 (setq ipl (polar f1i (* 1.5 pi ) (* 2 d) ) )
 (setq a1 0)
 (setq uzp ipl)
 (pldg)
 (setq uzp (polar ipl (* 0.5 pi ) d ) )
 (pldg)
 (setq num rnps)
 (setq uzp pls)
 (pldg)
 (setq uzp (polar pls (* 0.5 pi ) d ) )
 (pldg)
 (if (> hml oml )
 (progn
 (setq num rnpm)
 (setq uzp plm)
 (pldg)
 (setq g1 p2)
 (setq uzp (polar plm (* 0.5 pi ) d ) )
 (pldg)
 (setq g4 p4)
)
 (princ  "" )
)
(setq dx nplw dy d a1 (* 0.5 pi) )
 (setq num rnpw)
 (setq uzp (polar ipi 0 d) )
 (pldg)
 (setq uzp (polar ipi 0 (* 2 d) ) )
 (pldg)
 (setq num rnpe)
 (setq uzp (polar rvl1 0 d) )
 (pldg)
 (setq uzp rvl2 )
 (pldg)
 (opdg)
```

```
 (command "line" opm1 opm2 opm3 opm4 opm1 "" )
 (command)
)
(defun opdg ()
 (setq opm1 (polar g2 pi oml) )
 (setq opm4 (polar g3 pi oml) )
 (setq opm2 g2 opm3 g3)
 (command "line" opm1 opm4 "" )
 (setq ope1 (polar rvl3 (* 1.5 pi ) oel) )
 (setq ope4 (polar rvl4 (* 1.5 pi ) oel) )
 (setq ope2 rvl3 ope3 rvl4)
 (command "line" ope1 ope4 "" )
 (setq opw1 (polar opw3 (* 1.5 pi ) owl) )
 (setq opw2 (polar opw4 (* 1.5 pi ) owl) )
 (command "line" opw1 opw2 "" )
 (setq ops1 (polar ps1 pi osl) )
 (setq ops4 (polar ps2 pi osl) )
 (setq ops2 ps1 ops3 ps2)
 (command "line" ops1 ops4 "" )
 (setq opn1 (polar opn3 pi onl) )
 (setq opn2 (polar opn4 pi onl) )
 (command "line" opn1 opn2 "" )
 (setq pl1 (polar ipl 0 (* 0.5 nplw) ) )
 (setq pl2 (polar pl1 (* 0.5 pi) d ) )
 (setq pl3 (polar ipl (* 0.5 pi) (* 1.5 d ) ) )
 (setq pl4 (polar pl3 0 nplw) )
 (command)
)
(defun pldg ()
 (setq p1 uzp )
 (repeat num
 (dwof)
 (setq uzp p2)
)
 (command)
 )
(defun dwof ()
(setq p1 uzp)
(setq p2 (polar p1 a1 dx ) )
 (setq p3 (polar p1 (+ a1 (* 0.5 pi )) dy ))
 (setq p4 (polar p2 (+ a1 (* 0.5 pi )) dy ))
 (command "line" p1 p2 p4 p3 p1 "" )
)
(defun dwofb ()
 (setq p1 uzp )
 (setq p2 (polar p1 a1 dx ) )
 (setq p3 (polar p1 (+ a1 (* 0.5 pi )) dy ))
 (setq p4 (polar p2 (+ a1 (* 0.5 pi )) dy ))
```

```
(command "line" p1 p2 p4 p3 p1 "" )
)
(defun road ()
(setq dy 4 )
(prompt "\nroad offset length (in meter) is = " )
(princ (eval dy) )
(setq cofs (strcase (getstring "\ndo you want to change offset length ? (y/n): " )))
( if (= cofs "y")
(setq dy (getreal "\nenter desired offset length (changed)  : " ))
(princ   "" )
  )
(setq dx (- l (* 0.5 (+ m su) ) ) )
(setq uzp (list (car f1i ) (+ (cadr f1i) su dy) ) )
(setq a1 (* 1.5 pi ) )
(drgl)
(setq cornn p2 crne p3)
(setq dx (- b su) )
(setq uzp (list  (+ (car f2i) su dy) (cadr f2i ) ) )
(setq a1 pi )
(drgl)
(setq corne p2 )
(setq dx (- l (* 0.5 (+ m su) ) ) )
(setq uzp (list (car f0i ) (- (cadr f0i) (+ su dy )  )  ) )
(setq a1 (* 0.5 pi ) )
(drgl)
(setq corns p2 )
(setq dx (- b su) )
(setq uzp (list (- (car ipi) (+ m dy) ) (cadr ipi )  )  )
(setq a1 0 )
(drgl)
(setq cornw p2 )
(corner)
(rdtxt)
)
(defun drgl ()
(setq p1 uzp )
(setq p2 (polar p1 a1 dy ) )
(setq p3 (polar p2 (+ a1 (* 0.5 pi )) dx ) )
(setq p4 (polar p3 (+ a1 pi ) dy ) )
(command "line" p1 p2 p3 p4 "" )
)
(defun corner ()
(setq p2 (polar cornn pi m ) )
(setq dmm2 p2 )
(setq p1 (polar p2 (* 0.5 pi ) dy ) )
(setq p3 (polar p2 pi dy ) )
(command "line" p1 p2 p3 "" )
(setq p2 (polar corne (* 0.5 pi ) su ) )
```

```
 (setq dms2 p2 )
 (setq p1 (polar p2 (* 0.5 pi ) dy ) )
 (setq p3 (polar p2 0 dy ) )
 (command "line" p1 p2 p3 "" )
 (setq p2 (polar corns 0 su ) )
 (setq p1 (polar p2 (* 1.5 pi ) dy ) )
 (setq p3 (polar p2 0 dy ) )
 (command "line" p1 p2 p3 "" )
 (setq p2 (polar cornw (* 1.5 pi ) su ) )
 (setq p1 (polar p2 (* 1.5 pi ) dy ) )
 (setq p3 (polar p2 pi dy ) )
 (command "line" p1 p2 p3 "" )
)
(defun rdtxt ()
 (setq mtx  (list (- (car ipi) (* 0.1 m) ) (+ (cadr ipi) (* 0.5 (- b su) ) ) ) )
 (setq sntx (list (+ (car f1i) (* 0.5 (- l (* 0.5 (+ m su))))) (+ (cadr f1i) (* 0.1 su))))
 (setq setx (list (+ (car f0i) (* 0.9 su) ) (+ (cadr f0i) (* 0.5 (- b su) ) ) ) )
 (setq sstx (list (+ (car ipi) (* 0.5 (- l (* 0.5 (+ m su))))) (- (cadr ipi) (* 0.9 su) ) ) )
 (command "text" "c" mtx tx1 "90" "main road"
"text" "c" sntx tx1 "0" "subsidiary road"
"text" "c" setx tx1 "90" "subsidiary road"
"text" "c" sstx tx1 "0" "subsidiary road" )
 )
(defun txt ()
 (txsze)
 (command "text" "c"
 (list (+ (car f2) (* 24 tx1) ) (- (cadr f2) tx ) ) tx "0"
"HUDCO MODEL:-LAYOUT MODULE-A" )
 (setq cx1 (list (+ (car f2) (* 24 tx1) ) (- (cadr f2) (* 5 tx1 ) ) ) )
 (command "text" "c" cx1 tx1 "0"
"SOME INPUT-DESIGN-DECISIONS GIVEN"
"text" "c" (list (car cx1) (- (cadr cx1) (* 2 tx1 ) ) ) tx1 "0"
"TO SOFTWARE & CORRESPONDING"
"text" "c" (list (car cx1) (- (cadr cx1) (* 4 tx1 ) )  ) tx1 "0"
"OUTPUT-DESIGN-PARAMETER-VALUES"
"text" "c" (list (car cx1) (- (cadr cx1) (* 6 tx1 ) )  ) tx1 "0"
"GENERATED BY THE SOFTWARE :- " )
 (setq cx (list (+ (car f2) 10) (- (cadr f2) (* 16 tx2 ) ) ) )
 (command "text"
 (list  (car cx) (cadr cx)  )  tx2 "0"
"total land area (sq.m.) in layout module    ="
"text" (list (+ (car cx) tl) (cadr cx)  )  tx2 "0" stla
"text" (list (car cx ) (- (cadr cx) (* 2 tx2)  )   ) tx2 "0"
"total effective number of plots in module  ="
"text" (list (+ (car cx) tl) (- (cadr cx) (* 2 tx2)  ) ) tx2 "0" sn
"text" (list (car cx ) (- (cadr cx) (* 4 tx2)  )   ) tx2 "0"
"total blockwise number of full-size plots  ="
"text" (list (+ (car cx) tl) (- (cadr cx) (* 4 tx2)  ) ) tx2 "0" tnpl
```

```
"text" (list (car cx ) (- (cadr cx) (* 6 tx2) )  ) tx2 "0"
"length (e-w) of layout module (m)        ="
"text" (list (+ (car cx) tl) (- (cadr cx) (* 6 tx2) ) ) tx2 "0" sllyt
"text" (list (car cx ) (- (cadr cx) (* 8 tx2) )  ) tx2 "0"
"width (n-s) of layout module (m)         ="
"text" (list (+ (car cx) tl) (- (cadr cx) (* 8 tx2) ) ) tx2 "0" swlyt
"text" (list (car cx ) (- (cadr cx) (* 10 tx2) )  ) tx2 "0"
"given depth of plot (m)              ="
"text" (list (+ (car cx) tl) (- (cadr cx) (* 10 tx2) ) ) tx2 "0" spld
"text" (list (car cx ) (- (cadr cx) (* 12 tx2) )  ) tx2 "0"
"derived width of plot (m)             ="
"text" (list (+ (car cx) tl) (- (cadr cx) (* 12 tx2) ) ) tx2 "0" splw
"text" (list (car cx ) (- (cadr cx) (* 14 tx2) )  ) tx2 "0"
"gross cost of serviced land (mu/sq.m.)     ="
"text" (list (+ (car cx) tl) (- (cadr cx) (* 14 tx2) ) ) tx2 "0" sglc
"text" (list (car cx ) (- (cadr cx) (* 16 tx2) )  ) tx2 "0"
"market raw land price (mu/sq.m.)         ="
"text" (list (+ (car cx) tl) (- (cadr cx) (* 16 tx2) ) ) tx2 "0" slp
"text" (list (car cx ) (- (cadr cx) (* 18 tx2) )  ) tx2 "0"
"ratio of saleable land to layout area     ="
"text" (list (+ (car cx) tl) (- (cadr cx) (* 18 tx2) ) ) tx2 "0" sslr
"text" (list (car cx ) (- (cadr cx) (* 20 tx2) )  ) tx2 "0"
"ratio of circulation area to layout area   ="
"text" (list (+ (car cx) tl) (- (cadr cx) (* 20 tx2) ) ) tx2 "0" scirr
"text" (list (car cx ) (- (cadr cx) (* 22 tx2) )  ) tx2 "0"
"ratio of social-facility-area to layout area ="
"text" (list (+ (car cx) tl) (- (cadr cx) (* 22 tx2) ) ) tx2 "0" sspor
"text" (list (car cx ) (- (cadr cx) (* 24 tx2) )  ) tx2 "0"
"length of utility network per plot (m)     ="
"text" (list (+ (car cx) tl) (- (cadr cx) (* 24 tx2) ) ) tx2 "0" slut
"text" (list (car cx ) (- (cadr cx) (* 26 tx2) )  ) tx2 "0"
"plot density in layout (no.of plots/hectare) ="
"text" (list (+ (car cx) tl) (- (cadr cx) (* 26 tx2) ) ) tx2 "0" spden
"text" (list (car cx ) (- (cadr cx) (* 28 tx2) )  ) tx2 "0"
"given total affordable cost per plot (mu)  ="
"text" (list (+ (car cx) tl) (- (cadr cx) (* 28 tx2) ) ) tx2 "0" spc
"text" (list (car cx ) (- (cadr cx) (* 30 tx2) )  ) tx2 "0"
   "derived affordable area of plot (sq.m.)     ="
"text" (list (+ (car cx) tl) (- (cadr cx) (* 30 tx2) ) ) tx2 "0" spla )
 (setq d (list (car cx ) (- (cadr cx) (* 30 tx2) ) ) )
)
(defun paramtr ()
 (setq pden (* (/ n a) 10000) )
 (setq sl (/ (* n pa ) a ) )
 (setq glc (/ (* n pc) a ) )
 (setq li (/ (- (+ (* 2 l) (* 4 d) ) (+ m su) ) n ) )
 (setq ls (/ (+ l (* 0.5 b ) ) n ) )
 (setq lm (/ (* 0.5 b) n ) )
```

```
(setq lut (+ li ls lm ) )
(setq cirai (* (* (+ hl vl ) i ) 2 ) )
(setq ciras (- (+ (* l su) (* 0.5 su b ) ) (* 0.5 su su) ) )
(setq ciram (- (* 0.5 b m ) (* 0.5 m su) ) )
(setq cirr (/ (+ cirai ciras ciram ) a ) )
(setq spor (/ (* n o ) a ) )
(setq sllyt (rtos l 2 2 ))
(setq swlyt (rtos b 2 2 ))
(setq stla (rtos a 2 2 ))
(setq spla (rtos pa 2 2 ))
(setq splw (rtos nplw 2 2 ))
(setq spld (rtos d 2 2 ))
(setq sspo (rtos o 2 2 ))
(setq spden (rtos pden 2 2 ))
(setq sslr (rtos sl 2 2 ))
(setq scirr (rtos cirr 2 2 ))
(setq sspor (rtos spor 2 2 ))
(setq slp (rtos cl 2 2 ))
(setq sglc (rtos glc 2 2 ))
(setq slut (rtos lut 2 2 ))
(setq spc (rtos pc 2 2 ))
(setq sn (rtos n 2 2 ))
(setq sm (rtos m 2 2 ))
(setq ss (rtos su 2 2 ))
(setq si (rtos i 2 2 ))
)
(defun txsze ()
(setq tx 3.5 tx1 2.5 tx2 2.0 nx 45.0 )
(princ "\npre-set text-ht/loc.(k./nx)are:tx1=2.5,tx2=2.0,tx=3.5,nx=45.0 ")
(setq ctx ( strcase (getstring "\ndo you want to change the above values(y/n) ? " )))
(if (= ctx  "y" )
(progn
(setq tx1 (getreal "\nenter desired text ht.(tx1-heading)(changed)  : " ))
(setq tx2 (getreal "\nenter desired text ht.(tx2-general)  (changed)  : " ))
(setq tx  (getreal "\nenter desired text ht.(tx-top heading) (changed)  : " ))
(setq nx (getreal "\nenter desired text locn.(nx-mutiple data)(changed): " ))
)
(princ "" )
)
(setq tl (* nx tx2 ) )
)
(defun view ()
(setq vwdr (strcase ( getstring "\nyou want to change drawing view direction ? (y/n):")))
(while  (= vwdr "y" )
(setq ovwdr (strcase ( getstring "\ninsert existing output-drawing view direction
i(isometric)/p(plan) ? (i/p):")))
(setq ovwdrc (strcase ( getstring "\nyou want change of output-drawing view direction(i to p
,or, p to i ? (y/n):")))
```

```
(cond
((and (= ovwdr "i" ) (= ovwdrc "y" ) )
(command "vpoint" "r" "270.0" "90.0" )
)
((and (= ovwdr "p" ) (= ovwdrc "y" ) )
(progn
(command "vpoint" "r" "225.0" "30.0" )
(setq ciso (strcase ( getstring "\nyou want change iso-view direction from angle
30 to 45 ? (y/n):")))
(if (= ciso "y" )
(command "vpoint" "r" "225.0" "45.0" )
(princ "" )
)
)
)
)
(setq vwdr (strcase ( getstring "\nyou want to change drawing view direction ? (y/n):")))
)
)
(defun C:HUDCMOD ()
(command "limits" (list 0.0 0.0 ) (list 12.0 9.0 ) )
(command "zoom" "a" )
(prompt "\nWelcome to Design-Analysis-Drafting SOFTWARE for Layout-Module-A " )
(setq ersc ( strcase ( getstring "\nDo you want the Earlier Design(s) to be Erased(Y/N)? ")))
( if (= ersc "Y" )
(command "erase" ( ssget "x" ) "" )
(princ "" )
)
(lis2)
(lpar)
(command "zoom" "a" )
(setq ip (getpoint "\nput the drawing starting point (list) :   " ))
(setq ao 0 )
(setq f0 (list (+ (car ip) l ) (cadr ip) ) )
(setq f1 (polar ip (* 0.5 pi) b ) )
(setq f2 (polar f1 ao l) )
(setq ipi (list (+ (car ip) (* 0.5 m ) ) (+ (cadr ip) (* 0.5 su ) ) ) )
(setq f0i (list (- (car f0) (* 0.5 su ) ) (+ (cadr f0) (* 0.5 su ) ) ) )
(setq f1i (list (+ (car f1) (* 0.5 m ) ) (- (cadr f1) (* 0.5 su ) ) ) )
(setq f2i (list (- (car f2) (* 0.5 su ) ) (- (cadr f2) (* 0.5 su ) ) ) )
(setq uzp ipi)
(setq a1 0 )
(setq dx (* 2 d) )
(setq dy vl )
(dwofb)
(setq opw3 p3 opw4 p4 vb1 p1 vb2 p2)
(setq p1 (polar f0i (* 0.5 pi) (* 2 d) ) )
(setq p2 (polar p1 pi hl ) )
```

```
(setq p3 (polar f0i pi hl ) )
(setq pls p3 ps2 p1 ps1 f0i ps0 p2)
(setq ps3 (polar ps0 0 (* rnps nplw) ) )
(setq ps4 (polar pls 0 (* rnps nplw) ) )
(command "line" p1 p2 p3 f0i p1 "" )
(setq p1 (polar p2 (* 0.5 pi) i ) )
(setq plm p1 )
(setq p2 (polar p1 0 hml ) )
(setq p3 (polar p2 (* 0.5 pi) (* 2 d ) ) )
(setq p4 (polar p1 (* 0.5 pi) (* 2 d ) ) )
(setq plm1 p4 plm2 p2 plm3 p3)
(command "line" p1 p2 p3 p4 p1 "" )
(setq g2 p2 g3 p3)
(setq uzp f2i)
(setq a1 pi )
(setq dx (* 2 d) )
(setq dy vl )
(dwofb)
(setq rvl1 p4 rvl2 p3 rvl3 p2 rvl4 p1)
(setq p1 (polar f1i (* 1.5 pi) (* 2 d) ) )
(setq p2 (polar p1 0 hl ) )
(setq p3 (polar f1i 0 hl ) )
(command "line" p1 p2 p3 f1i p1 "" )
(setq opn3 p2 opn4 p3)
(plot)
(paramtr)
(command "linetype" "s" "continuous"  "" )
(command "line" ip f0 f2 f1 ip "c" )
(command "linetype" "s" "continuous"  "" )
(txt)
(road)
(dimen)
(command "zoom" "a" )
(view)\
)
```

In: Computer Graphics
Editor: Martin J. Davis
ISBN: 978-1-61761-811-6

Chapter 2

THE USE OF ADOBE PHOTOSHOP PROGRAM AS A PLANNING TOOL IN THE FIELD OF DEFORMITY CORRECTION SURGERY

Mohamed Kenawey[1,2], Emmanouil Liodakis[2], Mostafa Ismail[1], Christian Krettek[2], Anis Shiha[1] and Stefan Hankemeier[2]

[1]Orthopaedic Surgery Department, Sohag Faculty of Medicine, Sohag, Egypt
[2]Trauma Department, Hannover Medical School, Hannover, Germany

ABSTRACT

Digital preoperative planning is increasingly utilized in all fields of orthopaedic surgery. Reported advantages are higher accuracy, and reliability, time saving and digitally manipulating radiographs. On the other hand, high cost and unavailability are important limitations for their use. We would like to describe our experience with the use of one famous professional graphics editing programs, Adobe photoshop program, to plan our corrective surgeries in cases with deformities of the lower limbs.

In this work, we will describe the use of the Adobe photoshop program to correct a post-traumatic genu varus deformity through high tibial osteotomy. Our demonstrations will be limited to the principles of mechanical axis planning in the frontal plane and thereafter, different forms of valgus producing high tibial osteotomy to correct this post-traumatic varus deformity. The same principles can be used everywhere in a reasonably reproducible way.

Our demonstrations will be divided into the following areas:

I. Identify the source of deformity
    1. Mark the centers of hip, knee and ankle joints
    2. Mechanical axis and mechanical axis deviation (MAD)
    3. Joint orientation lines
    4. Joint orientation angles
II. Identify the level of the Center of Rotation of Angulation (CORA)
    1. Tibial mechanical axis planning

2. Femoral mechanical axis planning

III. Simulating corrective osteotomies
1. Open wedge osteotomy
2. Maquet dome osteotomy
3. Reversed focal dome osteotomy
4. Closing wedge osteotomy

Introduction

A preoperative plan is always needed before any deformity correction surgery in the lower extremities. Its methods were already described in a stepwise fashion to obtain reproducible results [1-4]. Lower limb deformities, and in particular those around the knee joint, are planned on long standing radiographs. This was usually performed manually using a pencil, long rulers and goniometer which is time consuming and its reliability cannot be always maintained [5].

On the other hand, computer assisted preoperative planning has become an essential part in many orthopaedic procedures [5,6]. Some commercial medical planning programs had been already developed and approved by the FDA (Food and Drug Administration) for use in the medical field [5,7]. The use of such specialized programs is limited by their cost and availability [6].

Reports describing the use of alternatives as professional graphics editing programs, in particular the Adobe Photoshop program, in the preoperative planning in many fields of orthopaedic surgery do exist [6,8,9]. Since 2007, the first author of this work (MK) started in his primary institution to develop methods to use the Adobe Photoshop program in the preoperative planning of deformity correction surgery. We have already described briefly our method [6], however the details of the steps of planning and in particular those of simulated corrective osteotomies and different types of complex osteotomies were not described.

The purpose of this work is to describe in a step by step fashion the details of the preoperative planning for corrective surgeries of lower extremity deformities using the Adobe photoshop program (version 10, Adobe System Incorporated, CA, USA). In the first part of this chapter, we will follow the description of Paley et al. [1-4] for the steps of mechanical axis planning in the frontal plane and how to define our deformity parameters as well as the level of the apex of the deformity or the CORA (Center of Rotation of Angulation). In the second part, we will describe in details the use of the program to simulate different types of corrective osteotomies.

Frontal Plane Mechanical Axis Planning

According to Paley et al. [1-4], mechanical axis planning in the frontal plane starts with the identification of the presence of malalignment (malalignment test) and to detect which type of malalignment and where the source is (femoral, tibial or combined deformities). The next step is to try to define the site of the apex of the deformity by defining the level of the CORA or CORAs within individual bony segments and their magnitude.

When an electronic version of our radiographs is opened using the Photoshop program, it will be considered as the first layer in a multi-layer image project. Any lines or text inserted in the next steps will be considered by the program as separate layers and therefore can be manipulated separately.

I. Identify the Source of Malalignment

To identify the source of a deformity, we should firstly check the mechanical axis of the lower limb. The mechanical axis of the whole limb is the line connecting the centers of the femoral head and the ankle joint, which in turn has a known relation to the center of the knee joint. This will give us an idea about the total alignment of the whole lower limb, whether it is normal or if there is a genu varus or valgus deformities. When the mechanical axis deviates medially or laterally outside its normal range, there will be a corresponding genu varus or valgus deformities respectively.

Therefore, the first step is to identify the central points of the hip joint (the center of the femoral head), the knee (we will use the midpoint of the femoral condyles and the midpoint of the tibial plateau for the femoral and tibial sides of the joint respectively) and the ankle joint (we prefer to use the midpoint between the medial and lateral shoulders of the talar dome).

In a next step, the mechanical axis of the lower limb will be drawn as well as other lines required for the mechanical axis planning. Line connecting the center of the femoral head to the midpoint of the femoral condyles and another line from the midpoint of the tibial plateau to the center of the ankle joint will be used to represent the mechanical axes of the femur and tibia respectively. These lines together with predefined joint orientation lines for hip, knee and ankle joints will allow for defining the orientation of each joint in relation to the mechanical axes and therefore concluding broadly if the source of deformity is mainly femoral, tibial or combined.

1. Mark The Centers Of The Hip, Knee And Ankle Joints

In order to mark the center of a specified area in a radiograph or an image, we should firstly select the outline of this area using the *Marquee tools*. The *Marquee (selection) tools* can be accessed from the *Tools*, stacked on the left side of the workspace [Keyboard shortcut *(M)*]. The *Elliptical Marquee tool* is used to mark elliptical selections. Holding the *Shift key* while we are using this tool makes a perfect circular selection (Figure 1). The *Rectangular Marquee tool* is used to mark rectangular areas (Figure 2 & 3).

The center of any selected area can be simply known by the *Free Transform (Ctrl + T)* command on the *Edit menu* (Figure 4). This command is used mainly to apply transformations (rotations, scaling, etc) to any selected area or selected layer inside an image. When chosen, a bounding box appears around the selection and a reference point will appear in the center of this bounding box. The cursor of the mouse can be stopped exactly over the reference point and then *Esc key* is pressed to cancel the transformation and the keyboard shortcut for the *Brush tool (B)* is used to mark this point.

By using this function with a circular selection which fits to the femoral head, we are identifying the femoral head center (Figure 4). To repeat these steps for the distal femur, proximal and distal tibial areas and the talar dome, the *Rectangular Marquee* is used. Using the rectangular selection tool in these areas will make selections which cannot fit the widest transverse diameter because of the obliquity of these planes from the horizontal plane. Therefore, right clicking the selection will display the shortcut menu including another option which is *Transform selection. Transform selection* can edit the shape of the selected areas without distorting the layer or the image itself as the case with the *Free Transform* command (Figure 2 & 3). We can use this option to rotate the rectangular selection for the best fit of the widest diameter of the anatomic area and to be in the same plane as the adjacent joint line. In the same time, while we are modifying the selection, the center is always displayed through the reference point.

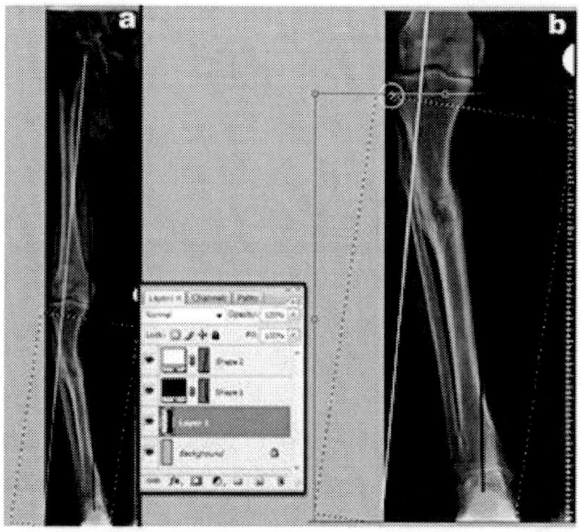

Figure 1. *Elliptical Marquee tool* from Tools is used mainly to mark elliptical and circular selections. The contour of the femoral head can be selected using this tool.

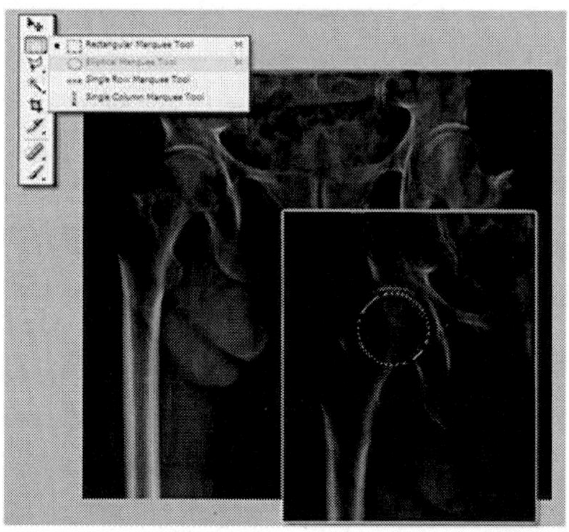

Figure 2. *Rectangular Marquee tool* can be used to mark rectangular selections in the distal femur and the orientations of these selections can be modified using *Transform Selection* from the shortcut menu which appears on right clicking the selected part (left). *Transform Selection* will also show the center of this selected area (right).

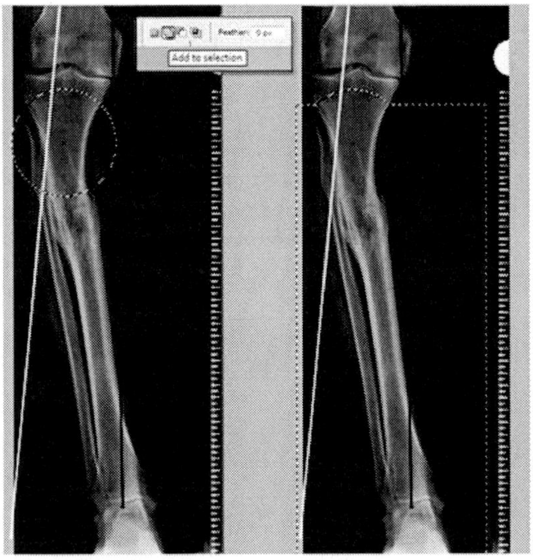

Figure 3. The same rectangular selections can be made in the proximal tibia (top left), distal tibial plafond (middle) and talar dome (bottom right).

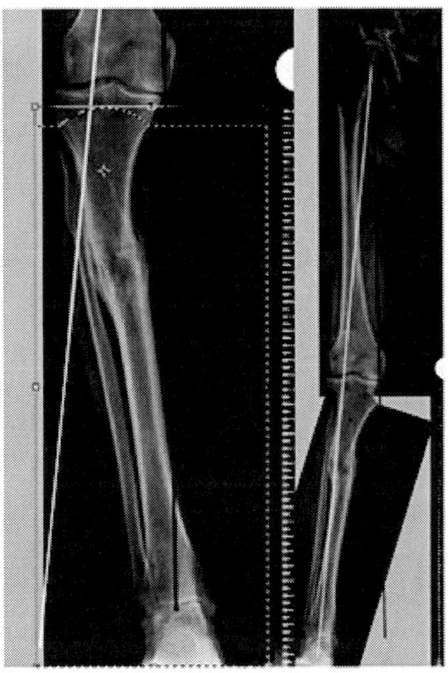

Figure 4. By using the *Free Transform option (Ctrl + T)* from *Edit menu*, a bounding box will appear around the selection and in this demonstration it appears around the circular selection of the contour of the femoral head with a reference point in the center of this selection. This center can be marked using the keyboard shortcut of the *Brush tool (B)*.

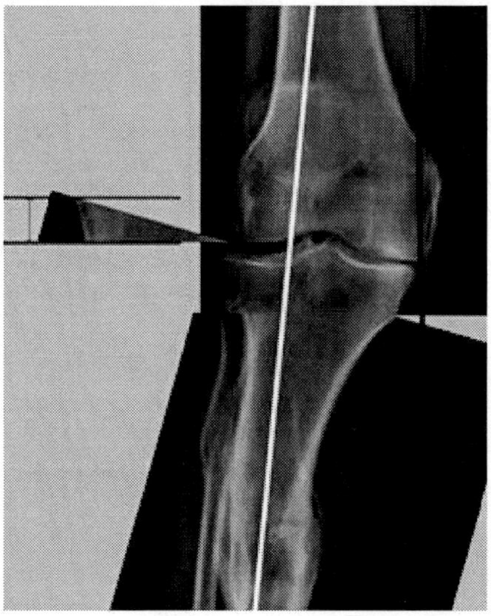

Figure 5. The mechanical axis of the whole extremity is drawn using the *Line tool (U)*. The distance between this line and the center of the knee joint can be measured using the *Ruler tool (I)* (right corner).

2. Mechanical Axis And MAD (Mechanical Axis Deviation)

With the *Line tool (U)*, a line is drawn between the centers of the femoral head and the ankle joint (the mechanical axis of the limb) (Figure 5). The *Ruler tool (I)* of the Adobe photoshop program can measure distances as well as angles. To measure the horizontal distance between the mechanical axis and the center of the knee joint (mechanical axis deviation), *Shift key* should be hold while we are using the ruler tool to make an exactly horizontal measurement line between both points. The measured distance will be displayed in the options toolbar, but it has no meaning by itself unless we know the magnification of the current radiograph. In the long standing lower limb radiographs, there is always a metallic sphere or any metallic marker of known diameter (here in our example there is both the metallic sphere 30 mm in diameter and a scale below it) (Figure 5). We can also measure the transverse diameter of the metallic sphere using the *Ruler tool* and then calculate the magnification factor and hence the mechanical axis deviation.

3. Joint Orientation Lines

The hip joint orientation line is the line drawn from the center of the femoral head to the tip of the greater trochanter (Figure 6). The knee joint orientation lines are the line for the distal femur connecting the two most convex points on the two femoral condyles and a line for the proximal tibia between the two most concave points of the medial and lateral tibial plateau (Figure 6). Regarding the ankle joint, we prefer a line across the flat subchondral bone of the tibial plafond. All of these lines can be simply drawn using the ***Line tool (U)***.

4. Joint Orientation Angles

Angles can be measured using the *Ruler tool (I)*. To measure any angle, we should firstly extend a measurement line from the apex of the angle to one limb. By holding the *Alt key* and moving the mouse cursor to the apex of the angle again, an angle sign will appear and another measurement line can now be extended from the apex to the other limb (Figure 7). The measured value will be displayed also on the options toolbar. Joint orientation angles of the lower extremity have unified nomenclature and known average values (Figure 8, Table 1).

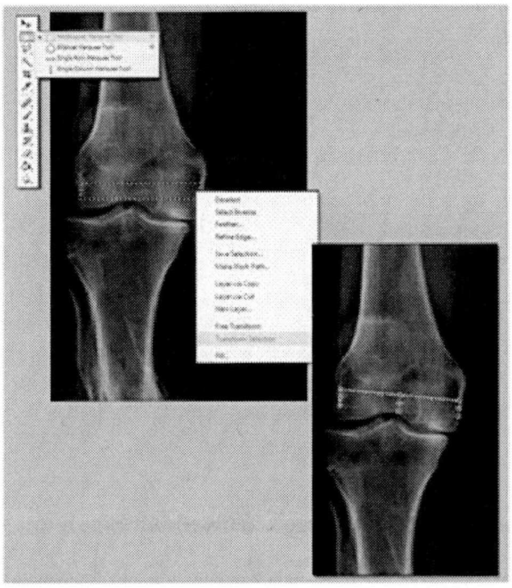

Figure 6. The joint orientation lines of the femoral head (top left), the knee joint (middle) and the ankle joint (bottom right) are drawn using the *Line tool.*

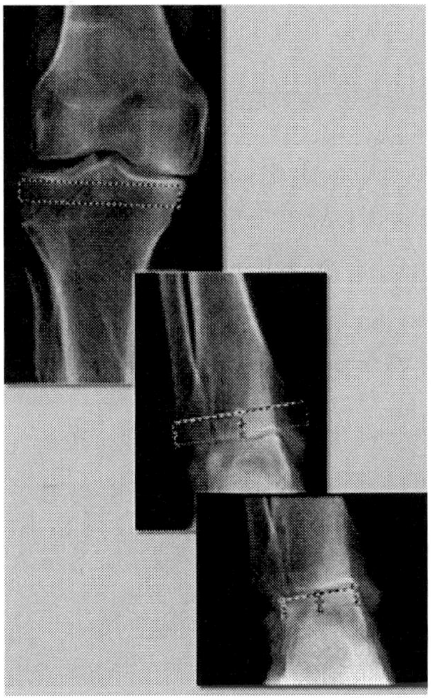

Figure 7. Measurement of angles is accomplished using the *Ruler tool (I)* and the measured value is displayed in the *Options toolbar* next to the angle sign (highlighted area). In this demonstration the angle is 87.3°.

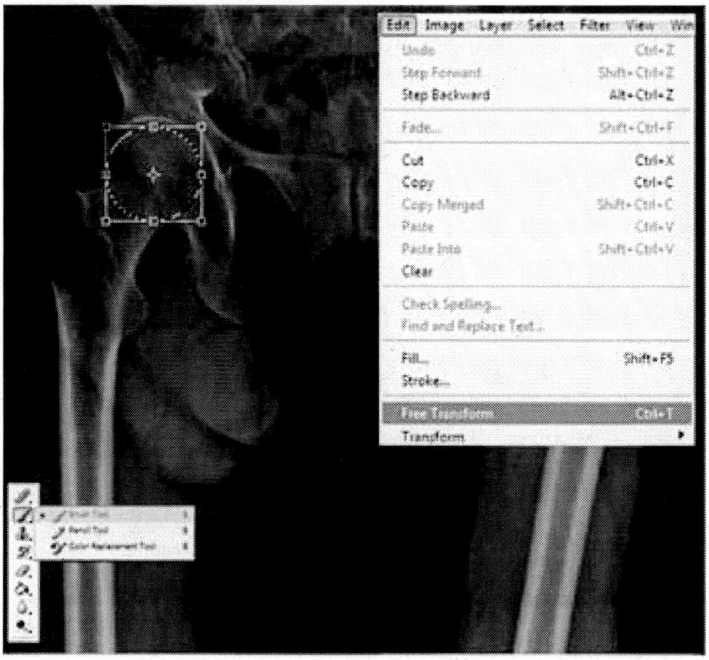

Figure 8. Different joint orientation angles can be measured and abnormal values will indicate an abnormality in this bony segment.

Table 1. Joint orientation angles, definitions and average values (range), used in mechanical axis planning in the frontal plane of the lower extremities.

LPFA	Lateral Proximal Femoral Angle The angle between the femoral mechanical axis and the line connecting the center of the femoral head with the tip of the greater trochanter	90° (85 – 95°)
mLDFA	mechanical Lateral Distal Femoral Angle The angle between the femoral mechanical axis and the distal femoral orientation line	88° (85 – 90°)
JLCA	Joint Line Convergence Angle The angle between distal femoral and proximal tibial orientation lines	0 – 2°
MPTA	Medial Proximal Tibial Angle The angle between proximal tibial orientation line and the tibial mechanical axis.	87° (85 – 90°)
LDTA	Lateral Distal Tibial Angle The angle between the tibial mechanical axis and the ankle joint orientation line	90° (86 – 92°)

II. Identify the Level of the CORA

The next step in the process of defining the deformity parameters should be the identification of the apex of the deformity. To detect the deformity apex, each bony segment will be divided into proximal and distal parts and the mechanical and anatomical axes of each part can be drawn separately. The point of intersection of the lines representing axes of the proximal and the distal segments is called the center of rotation of angulation (CORA) [1]. The angle measured at the CORA is the magnitude of our deformity.

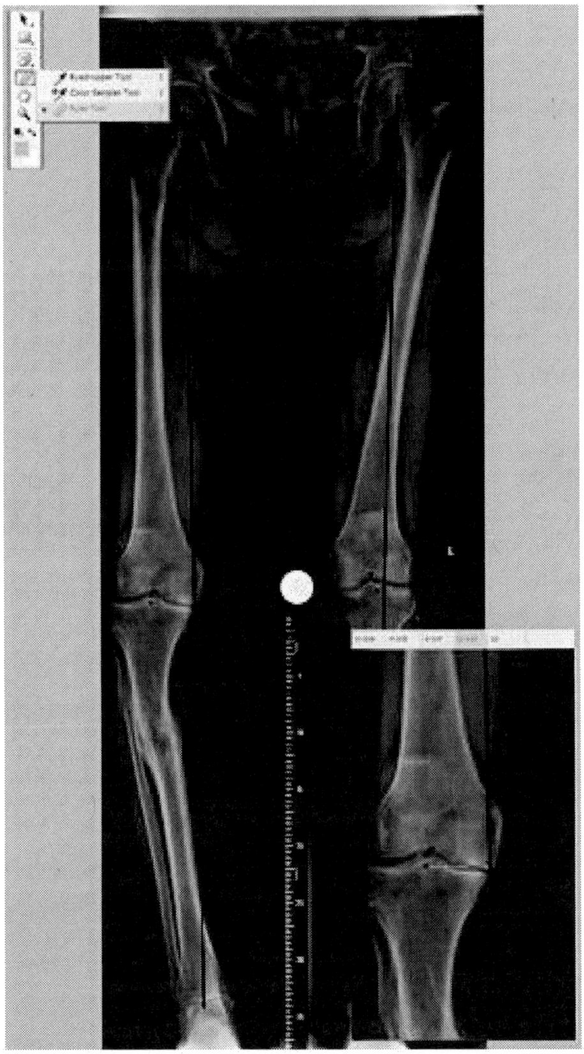

Figure 9. Right clicking the layer which represents the proximal tibial orientation line *(Shape 1)* in this example will give up the shortcut menu and this menu contains the *Duplicate Layer* choice (the highlighted choice). Clicking this choice will duplicate the mentioned layer and a secondary window will appear with the options of this command like the name which we would choose for this new layer and by default will be *(Shape 1 copy)*.

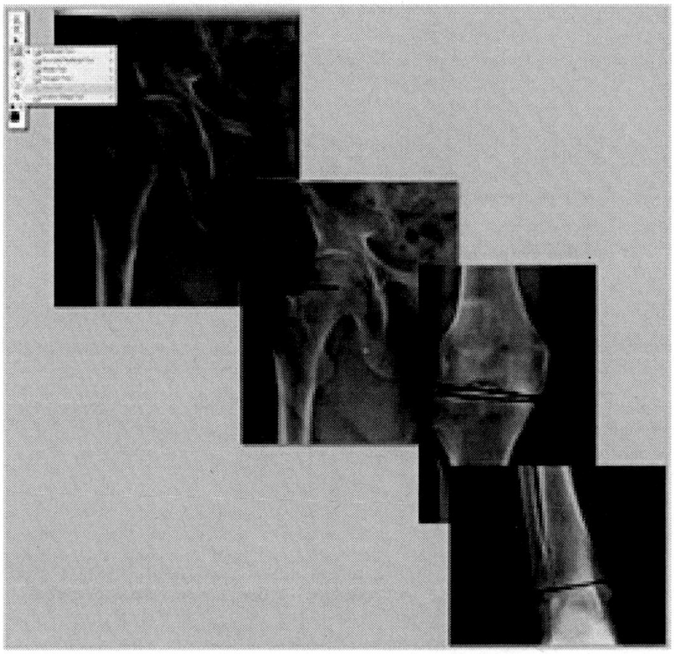

Figure 10. Choose the new duplicate layer (*shape 1 copy*) and then from the Edit menu, the *Free Transform Path (Ctrl + T)* option is used to rotate this layer or that line.

1. Tibial Mechanical Axis Planning

To draw the proximal tibial mechanical axis, a line should be drawn with a specific angle to the proximal tibial orientation line. This angle is equal to the MPTA (Medial Proximal Tibial Angle) obtained from the healthy side or the average value (87°). By right clicking the layer which represents the proximal tibial orientation line, this layer can be duplicated using the *Duplicate layer* choice from the corresponding shortcut menu (Figure 9). Then the new duplicate layer can be rotated using the Free Transform Path from the Edit menu (Ctrl + T) (Figure 10). This rotation can be done using the mouse or by typing the value of 87° directly in the options toolbar in the section with the angle sign (Figure 11). The new line is then moved to start from the midpoint of the tibial plateau (Figure 12).

The distal tibial mechanical axis is a line which is parallel to the tibial anatomical axis, but starts from the center of the ankle joint. The tibial anatomical axis is the mid-diaphyseal line (the line connecting mid-diaphyseal points). Using the same principles by which we have marked the centers of the knee and ankle joints, rectangular selections are done within the shaft area (diaphysis) of the tibial bone. Two mid-diaphyseal points are marked using these selections and the line which connects these two points is the anatomical axis of the tibia. We can then move this line to get a starting point from the ankle center and to become the distal tibial mechanical axis (Figure 13). The point of intersection of the two lines (the proximal and distal tibial mechanical axes) is the CORA or the apex of the deformity. The magnitude of the deformity at this apex can be measured directly by measuring the angle between the two lines (Figure 14).

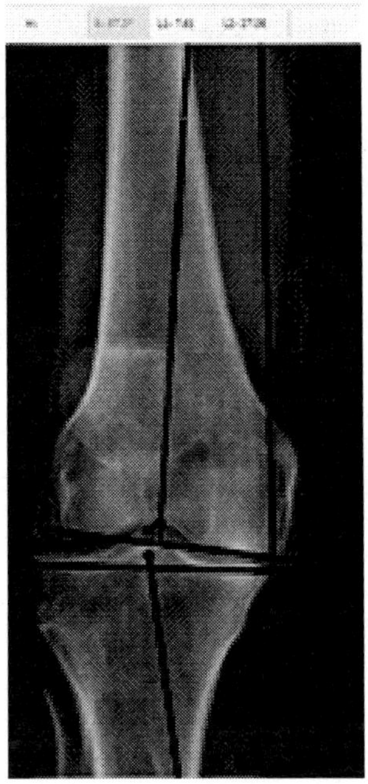

Figure 11. Rotating any layer with the Free Transform command is done using directly the mouse with the free hand or by typing the value of the angle in the options toolbar within the section just next to the angle sign (the highlighted section).

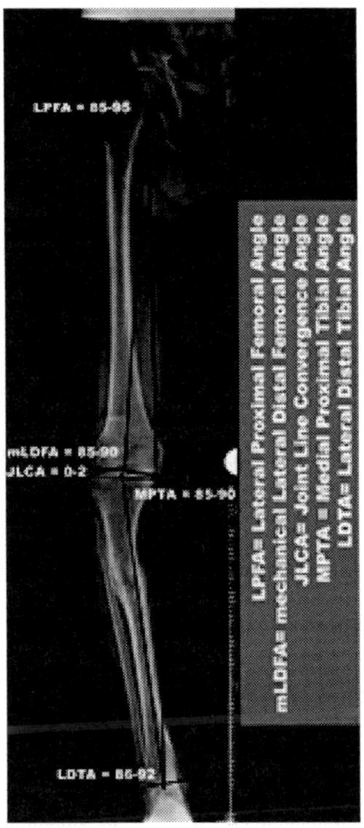

Figure 12. After rotating the layer, it can be simply dragged till the line comes in contact with the center of the tibial plateau to become the proximal tibial mechanical axis.

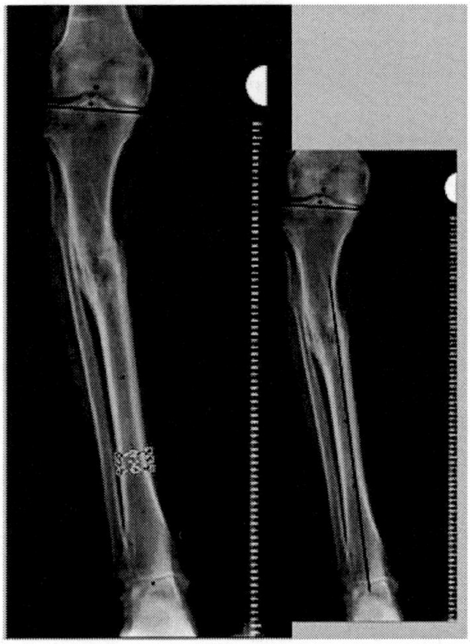

Figure 13. By marking rectangular areas within the shaft of the tibia (left image) and then defining the centers of these selections, we are defining mid-diaphyseal points. The line which connects these mid-diaphyseal points is the tibial anatomical aixs which can be moved to the center of the ankle joint to be the distal tibial mechanical axis (right image).

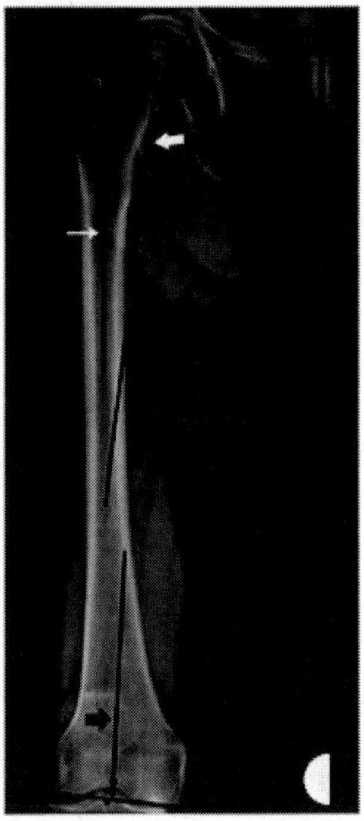

Figure 14. The intersection of the proximal and distal tibial mechanical axes is the point of the deformity apex or the CORA (the black arrow). The angle between both lines is the magnitude of this deformity.

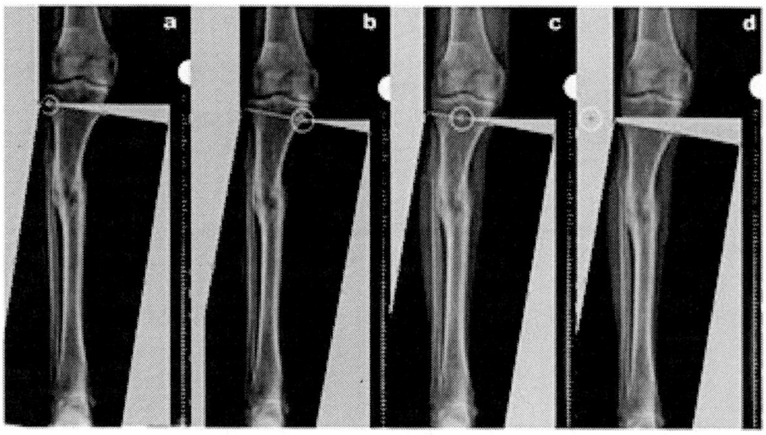

Figure 15. This femoral radiograph shows the distal femoral mechanical axis starting from the center of the femoral condyles (black arrow), the femoral anatomical axis (white thin arrow) and the proximal femoral mechanical axis which starts from the center of the femoral head and is drawn in reference to the anatomical axis (white thick arrow). Here we see that the proximal and distal mechanical axes are nearly parallel and therefore no deformity is present in the femoral side of the lower extremity.

2. Femoral Mechanical Axis Planning

The distal femoral mechanical axis is drawn using the same steps described for the proximal tibial mechanical axis. This distal femoral mechanical axis replicates the normal mLDFA (mechanical Lateral Distal Femoral Angle) of the normal side or uses an average adult value (88°) (Figure 15). On the other side, the proximal femoral mechanical axis is drawn with reference to the femoral anatomical axis. Unlike the tibia where the anatomical and mechanical axes are parallel, there is an angle between the femoral anatomical and mechanical axes which in average 7° (the anatomical mechanical angle; AMA). Therefore, the anatomical axis of the proximal shaft area of the femur can be drawn and then duplicated and rotated by about 7° and moved to start from the center of the femoral head (Figure 15).

III. Simulating Corrective Osteotomies

One of the main advantages of the Adobe photoshop program is the wide variability of options that allow for large deal of freedom in manipulating images. We can simply select part of our radiograph which in turn can be separately manipulated using the *Free Transform*. Furthermore, the reference point of such transformations acts as a center for the rotation and scaling functions. This reference point can be moved freely anywhere inside the image, modifying accordingly the center of our rotation which is known in deformity correction surgery as ACA (Angulation correction axis). As an example, in case of valgus producing high tibial osteotomy, moving the rotation center to the medial cortex of the tibia at the same level of an osteotomy will result in a closing wedge osteotomy while if moved to the lateral cortex will produce an open wedge osteotomy and in between both cortices, a neutral wedge osteotomy will be the result. We can manipulate our selected part freely to test the different concepts of osteotomies described by Paley et al. [1] and to see the resulting displacements and distractions and to have a clear idea about the final result of our corrective procedure; if executed as planned (Figure 16).

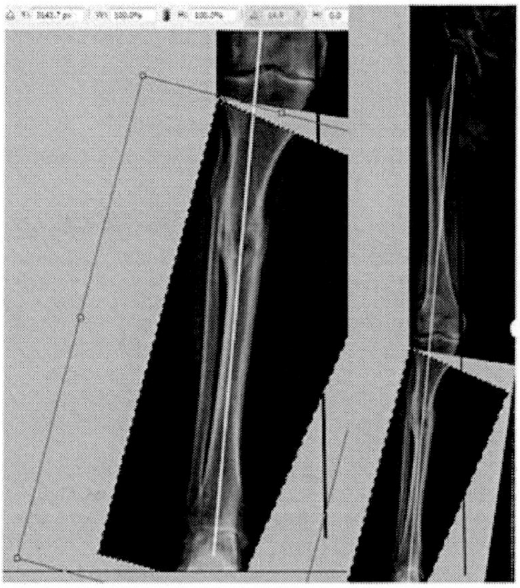

Figure 16. Moving the reference point of the *Free Transforms* (the white circle) will move accordingly the center of rotation of this part within the selection area. In the current example, we will try to modify the center of rotation of a valgus producing high tibial transverse osteotomy. a: If the reference point is located at the lateral tibial cortex at the same level of the proximal end of the selection (which represents the line of the osteotomy), a pure open wedge osteotomy will be made. b: closing wedge osteotomy is produced by a reference point at the medial tibial cortex. c: neutral wedge osteotomy can be produced by a reference point in between the medial and lateral tibial cortices. d: open wedge correction with lengthening (distraction) will be the result of a reference point located laterally away from the tibial cortex but at the same level of osteotomy.

1. Open Wedge Osteotomy

In our demonstrations, we will simulate a medial open wedge, valgus producing high tibial osteotomy to correct a post-traumatic varus deformity. We will use the modification described by Lobenhoffer and Agneskirchner [10] with an oblique medial open wedge ostetomy which runs from distal medial to proximal lateral (starting from the upper border of the pes anserinus tendons and ending nearly at the level of the fibular head). To calculate the amount of required correction, we will use the method described by Murphy [11].

Firstly, a line is drawn from the center of the femoral head passing through the desired point on the tibial plateau (Fujisawa point) (Figure 17). At this point, the weight-bearing axis should intersect with the knee joint line at 60-70% of the tibial plateau entire width measured from the medial cortex [12]. A rectangular selection is made starting from the level of the proposed osteotomy till the distal end of the radiograph. Then the *Transform selection* is used to rotate the selection so that its upper border takes the same level and orientation of the planned osteotomy as described by Lobehoffer and Agneskirchner [10] (Figure 17).

The ***Free Transform*** is then chosen and its reference point is moved to the lateral tibial cortex at the same level of the osteotomy to give a pure open wedge osteotomy (Figure 17). The selected part is now rotated freely around this new center of rotation until the center of the ankle joint lies on the corrected mechanical axis which passes through Fujisawa point (Figure 18). The final result will be a corrected limb with a new mechanical axis which passes through the lateral tibiofemoral compartment. Magnitude of correction is displayed at the options toolbar in the form of degrees of rotation required to get the center of the ankle joint on the new mechanical axis (Figure 18). An additional useful step is to measure the length of the base of the open wedge, which is useful during the intraoperative execution of the osteotomy.

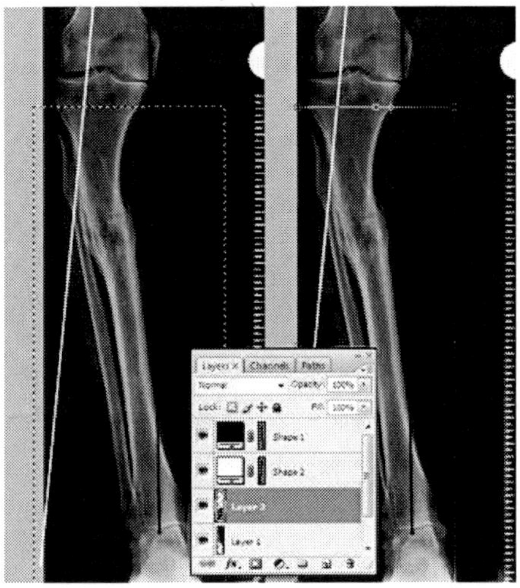

Figure 17. The method described by Murphy for calculating the magnitude of correction through high tibial osteotomy is demonstrated in this example. a: the first step is to extend a line (the white line) from the center of the femoral head passing through the lateral tibial plateau at Fujisawa point for example. Then area starting from the proximal tibia at the level of proposed osteotomy till the inferior end of the radiograph is selected using the rectangular selection tool and this selection is modified till its upper border lies at the same level of the proximal tibial osteotomy and takes the same orientation. b: the *Free Transform* option is used and the reference point is moved to the point at which the upper border of the rectangular selection cuts the lateral tibial cortex the white circle.

2. Maquet Dome Osteotomy

The original barrel vault or dome osteotomy was described by Maquet [13]. This osteotomy is dome shaped, made above the tibial tuberosity to take the advantage of better healing characteristics of the cancellous area with its concavity directed distally. This makes its center of rotation distal to the tibial tuberosity. To simulate this osteotomy type, the combination of *Elliptical Marquee tool* + *Shift Key* is used to make a circular selection with its proximal border at the proposed level of the osteotomy. Using the *Transform selection*, the center of this circle is marked on the tibia. In the *Options toolbar*, general options for selections are displayed and we should now choose *Add to selection* (Figure 19). Now, *Rectangular Marquee tool* is used to add a rectangular selection to the existing circular one. The rectangular selection should start proximally at the level where the proximal part of the circular selection (which simulates the osteotomy) cuts the medial and lateral tibial cortices and extends distally to the end of the radiograph (Figure 19).

The next steps are similar to what was done to simulate an open wedge osteotomy. *Free Transform* is used and the reference center is moved to the previously marked center of the first circular selection which will be the rotation center for the dome osteotomy. Correction is performed till the center of the ankle lies on the corrected mechanical axis and the magnitude of correction is recorded from the angle section in the *Options toolbar* (Figure 20).

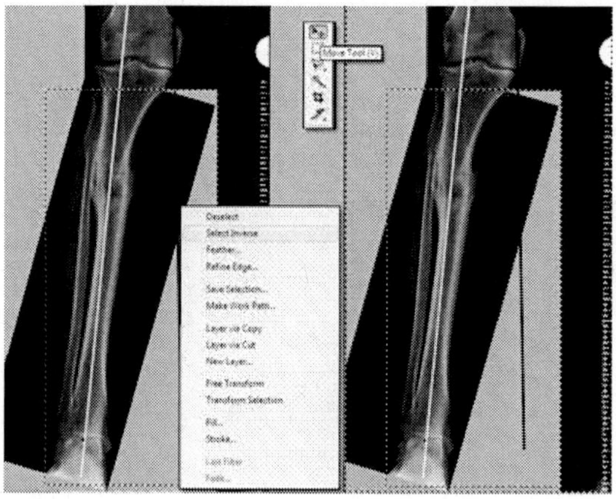

Figure 18. The selected part of the radiograph is rotated until the center of the ankle joint lies on the corrected mechanical axis (White line). The magnitude of this correction is displayed in the options toolbar in the section next to the angle sign which is 14.9° in this example (Highlighted).

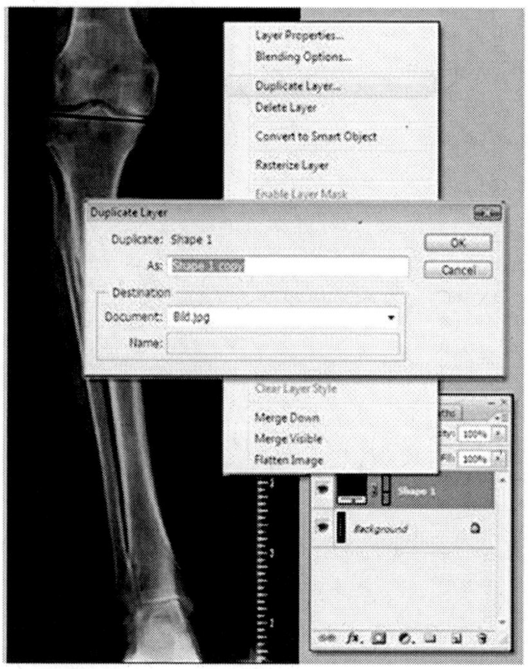

Figure 19. To simulate Maquet dome osteotomy, a perfect circle is selected in the area of the proximal tibia with its upper border at the same site and have the same orientation of the proposed osteotomy (left). The center of this circle is marked (black dot) and then selecting the *Add to selection* option from the options toolbar. When a rectangular selection is made with its proximal end at the level where the proximal part of the previous circular selection cuts the tibial cortices, the result will be as displayed in the right part of the figure.

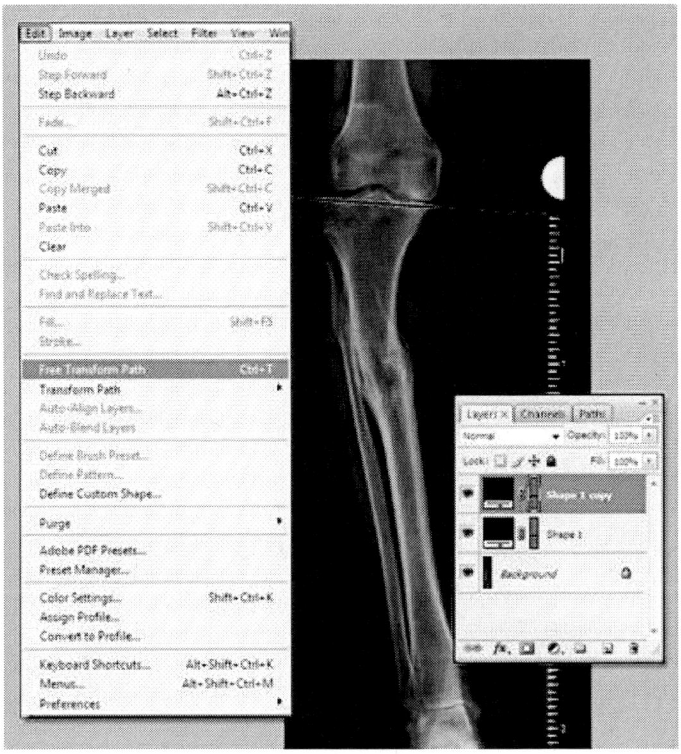

Figure 20. The same as the previous example for open wedge osteotomy, the *Free Transform* command is used and the reference point is moved to the previously marked center of the circular selection (left). The selected part is rotated till the center of the ankle joint lies on the corrected mechanical axis (right).

3. Reversed Focal Dome Osteotomy

Reversed focal dome osteotomy was described with the main osteotomy line distal to the tibial tuberosity but its concavity is directed proximally which is the reverse in relation to Maquet osteotomy [1,14]. This modification made the center of the dome and hence its center of rotation lying proximally near the joint line. In fact, it is an important modification because most patients with varus knees and medial compartment osteoarthritis have the apex of deformity near the joint line and therefore it is beneficial to make the ACA also near the deformity apex.

A perfect circular selection is made using the combination *Shift key + Elliptical Marquee tool* with its center near the knee joint line. The distal border of the circle should simulate the osteotomy line in level and orientation and the center of this circle is then marked on the radiograph (Figure 21). Right clicking the selection and then choosing *Layer via cut* from the corresponding shortcut menu will cut this circular part of from the layer of the radiograph and will make a new layer with this part. From the Layers, we choose the layer representing the remaining part of the long standing radiograph. A rectangular selection is made from the level of the osteotomy extending to the distal end of the radiograph (Figure 22).

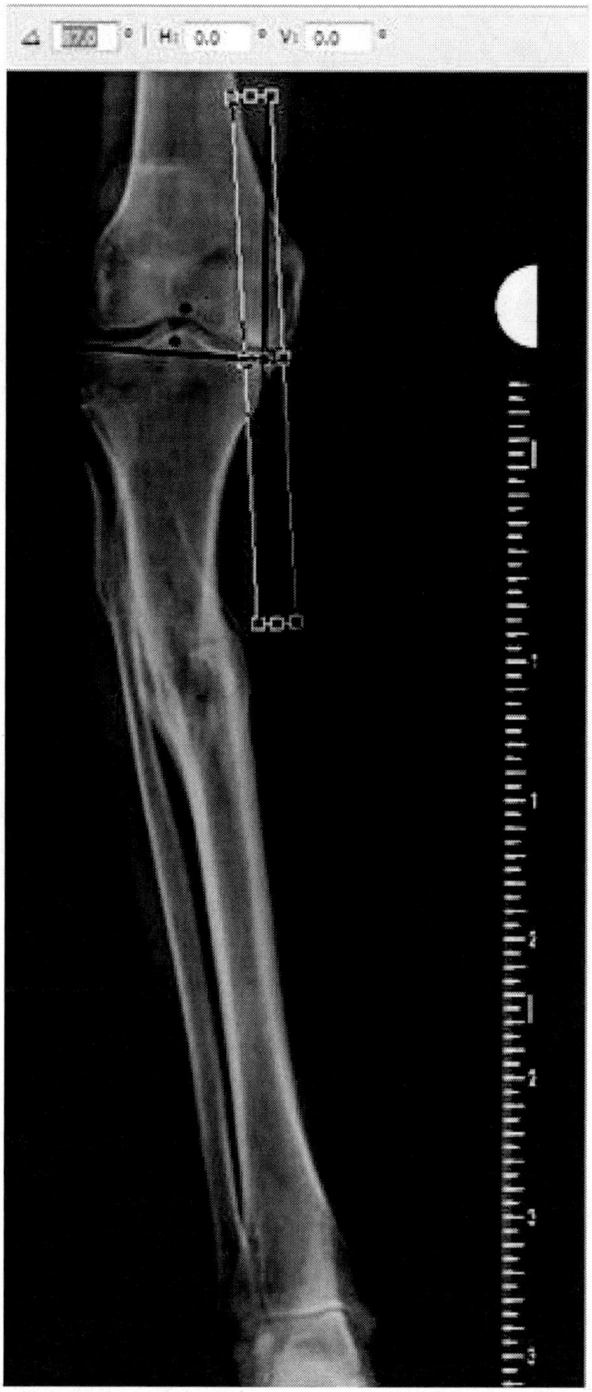

Figure 21. The main idea when simulating the reversed focal dome osteotomy is to make a perfect circular selection within the layer of the original radiograph (in this demonstration it is *Layer 1*) with its distal border representing the osteotomy line. By right clicking the selection, we choose *Layer via Cut* option (left). This will cut the selected circular part and will consider it a new layer (*Layer 2*).

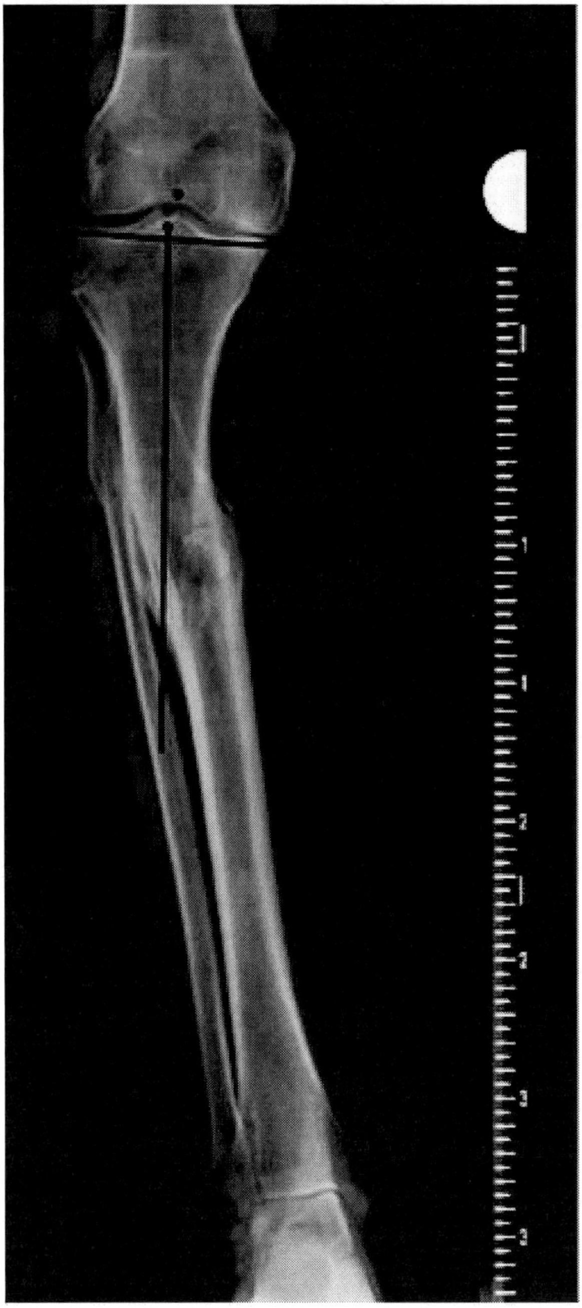

Figure 22. A rectangular selection is then chosen within *Layer 1* from the level of the osteotomy distalwards (left). This selection is then rotated till the center of the ankle lies on the corrected mechanical axis (right).

Similar to the previously described sequences of correction, the *Free Transform* command is chosen and then the reference center is moved to the previously marked center of the circular selection. The deformity is corrected as described previously and the magnitude of correction is then recorded (Figure 22).

4. Closing Wedge Osteotomy

The most important step in planning of closing wedge osteotomies is the measurement of the height of the wedge base to be resected. The remaining steps are similar to that of open wedge osteotomy. A rectangular selection is made starting from the level of the proposed osteotomy to the distal end of the radiograph. This selected part is cut as a new layer by the *Layer via Cut* option and then this new layer is rotated with the reference point of the *Free Transform* at the medial tibial cortex (Figure 23). Correcting the deformity till the center of the ankle lies on the corrected mechanical axis will be accomplished through overlapping the lateral cortices of the proximal and distal tibial fragments (Figure 24). While the layer representing the distal part of the tibia is still chosen, a rectangular selection is then made replicating the previous one, in particular regarding its proximal level. The *Select inverse* choice can be used to inverse this selection, therefore the area outside this rectangle will be actively selected. This in turn will select the wedge which overlapped the proximal part of the tibia. This wedge can be moved away and the height of its base measured (Figure 25).

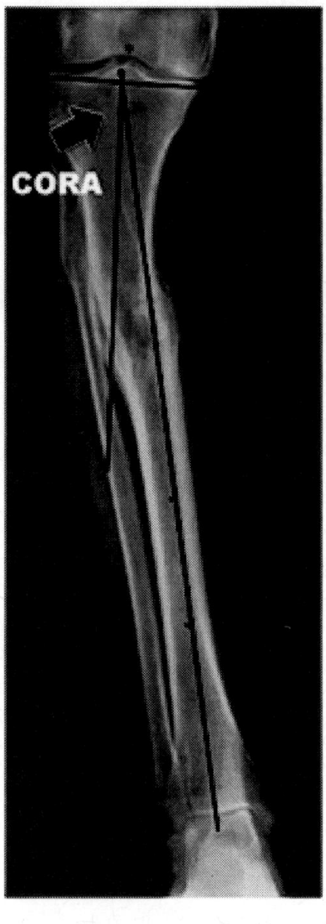

Figure 23. For closing wedge osteotomies, a rectangular selection is made from the level of the proposed osteotomy to the distal end (left) and then cut as a new layer (*Layer 2*). This new layer is chosen in the *Layers* and rotated using *Free Transform* while its reference point at the medial tibial cortex (right).

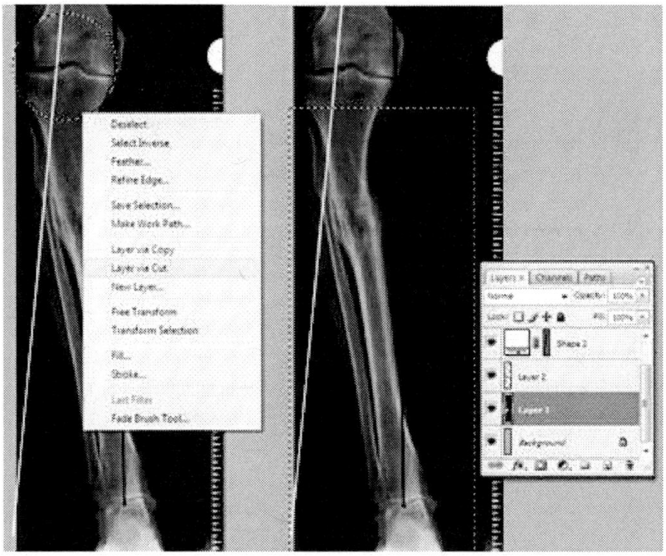

Figure 24. After correction the lateral cortices from both layers representing the distal and proximal parts of the tibia are overlapped. We should now make a rectangular selection replicating the previously selected one in Figure 23. With *Select inverse* option we can select the part of the distal tibia outside this rectangle which will be the wedge of the osteotomy.

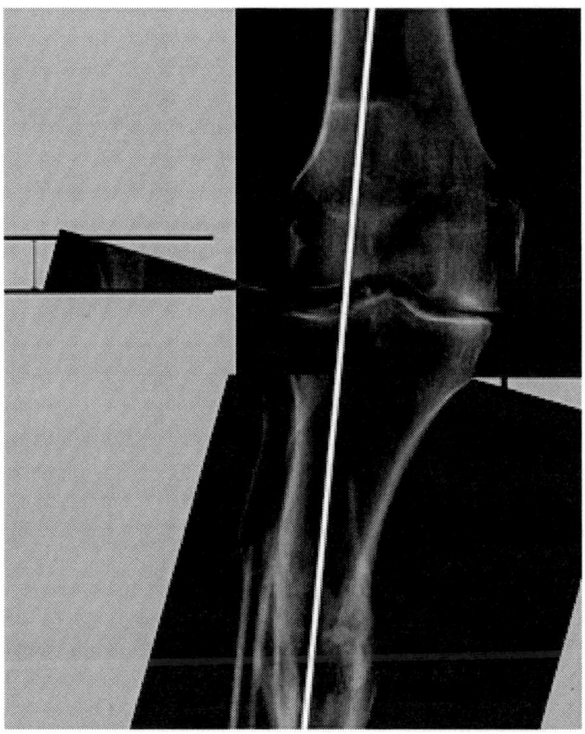

Figure 25. This selected wedge can be moved using the ***Move tool*** and the height of its base measured.

CONCLUSION

The current work shows clearly that the use of professional graphics editing programs can be extended to include highly specialized areas in the medical field. The advantages of using the Adobe Photoshop program in the preoperative planning of deformity correction surgery are mainly related to the large degree of freedom to manipulate our pictures and radiographs. We are not limited with specific functions or commands performing specific tasks. This gives the chance to be creative; trying new ideas, changing the shapes of our osteotomies and manipulating centers of rotations. Furthermore, general options as the control of the image format, resolution and color channel can be easily accessed.

We think also that the current work provides the basics of the general use of such programs and the basic concepts of managing layers, using tools and options which can be extended everywhere and with every type of graphics. Lastly, professional graphics editing programs are very good alternatives for specialized medical software in the field of computer assisted preoperative planning in orthopaedic surgery.

CONFLICT OF INTEREST STATEMENT

None of the authors have any commercial associations (e.g., consultancies, stock ownership, equity interest, patent/licensing arrangement, etc.) that might pose a conflict of interest in connection with the submitted article. There was no financial support for this study.

REFERENCES

[1] Paley, D. Principles of deformity correction. *Springer-Verlag, Berlin, Heidelberg, New York. 1st Edition*, 2002.

[2] Paley, D; Herzenberg, JE; Tetsworth, K; McKie, J; Bhave, A. Deformity planning for frontal and sagittal plane corrective osteotomies. *Orthop Clin North Am.*, 1994, 25-3, 425-65.

[3] Paley, D; Tetsworth, K. Mechanical axis deviation of the lower limbs. Preoperative planning of multiapical frontal plane angular and bowing deformities of the femur and tibia. *Clin Orthop Relat Res.*, 1992-280, 65-71.

[4] Paley, D; Tetsworth, K. Mechanical axis deviation of the lower limbs. Preoperative planning of uniapical angular deformities of the tibia or femur. *Clin Orthop Relat Res.*, 1992-280, 48-64.

[5] Hankemeier, S; Gosling, T; Richter, M; Hufner, T; Hochhausen, C; Krettek, C. Computer-assisted analysis of lower limb geometry: higher intraobserver reliability compared to conventional method. *Comput Aided Surg.*, 2006, 11-2, 81-6.

[6] Shiha, A; Krettek, C; Hankemeier, S; Liodakis, E; Kenawey, M. The use of a professional graphics editing program for the preoperative planning in deformity correction surgery: A technical note. *Injury*, 2009.

[7] Trickett, RW; Hodgson, P; Forster, MC; Robertson, A. The reliability and accuracy of digital templating in total knee replacement. *J Bone Joint Surg Br*, 2009, 91-7, 903-6.

[8] Gong, HS; Chung, MS; Oh, JH; Cho, HE; Baek, GH. Oblique closing wedge osteotomy and lateral plating for cubitus varus in adults. *Clin Orthop Relat Res.*, 2008, 466-4, 899-906.
[9] Jamali, AA. Digital templating and preoperative deformity analysis with standard imaging software. *Clin Orthop Relat Res.*, 2009, 467-10, 2695-704.
[10] Lobenhoffer, P; Agneskirchner, JD. Improvements in surgical technique of valgus high tibial osteotomy. *Knee Surg Sports Traumatol Arthrosc*, 2003,11-3, 132-8.
[11] Murphy, SB. Tibial osteotomy for genu varum. Indications, preoperative planning, and technique. *Orthop Clin North Am.*, 1994, 25-3, 477-82.
[12] Fujisawa, Y; Masuhara, K; Shiomi, S. The effect of high tibial osteotomy on osteoarthritis of the knee. An arthroscopic study of 54 knee joints. *Orthop Clin North Am*, 1979,10-3, 585-608.
[13] Maquet, P. Valgus osteotomy for osteoarthritis of the knee. *Clin Orthop Relat Res.*, 1976-120, 143-8.
[14] Hankemeier, S; Paley, D; Pape, HC; Zeichen, J; Gosling, T; Krettek, C. [Knee para-articular focal dome osteotomy]. *Orthopade*, 2004, 33-2,170-7.

In: Computer Graphics
Editor: Martin J. Davis

ISBN: 978-1-61761-811-6

Chapter 3

COMPUTER GRAPHICS AND MEDICAL IMAGE PROCESSING IN A SURGICAL NAVIGATION SYSTEM FOR ORAL AND MAXILLOFACIAL SURGERY

Chen Xiaojun[1]

[1] Institute of Biomedical Manufacturing and Life Quality Engineering, School of Mechanical Engineering, Shanghai Jiao Tong University, Shanghai, China

ABSTRACT

Surgical procedures in the cranio-maxillofacial region require a detailed knowledge of this region's complex anatomy. The limited intraoperative visibility, especially the anatomical intricacies, makes this kind of surgery a demanding procedure. Due to the expanding application of computer technology in medicine, new methods are evolving for medical diagnosis and presurgical planning, and especially for guiding or performing surgical interventions. Nowadays, computer-assisted navigation technology has become almost routine in neurosurgery. However, in the field of oral and maxillofacial surgery, these neurosurgery-oriented navigation systems had to be adapted and the software changed, especially with respect to preoperative planning, where more complicated algorithms in computer graphics and medical image processing are involved.

This study presents an image guided system for oral and maxillofacial surgery, which integrates 3D medical modeling, preoperative surgical planning and intraoperative tracking into a surgical navigation system. With the aid of this system, the precision achieved in the planning phase can be transferred to the operating theatre so that the feasibility and reliability of oral and maxillofacial surgery can be achieved in anatomically complex operation sites. Various algorithms in the field of computer graphics and medical image processing are involved in this system, including DICOM file parsing, image segmentation and 3D-visualization, surface decimation, cutting, collision detection, spatial search and 3D distance computing, volume measurement, spline curve generation, boolean operation, multi(curved)-planar reconstruction, image registration, etc. For each of these algorithms, a set of dynamic link libraries (DLL) were developed using C++, as well as the VTK and ITK via object oriented programming methodology. Therefore, a plug-in evolutive architecture was established, allowing for expandability, accessibility, and maintainability in our system. Benefits of the preoperative planning software, as well as this navigation system, are demonstrated in the clinical cases of oral and maxillofacial surgery, ranging from dental implantology to as far as the treatment of craniofacial malformations and advanced tumours within this anatomically complex region.

Keywords: Computer graphics, Medical image processing, Computer-aided oral and maxillofacial surgery, Surgical navigation

I. Introduction

Oral and maxillofacial surgery is surgery to treat the entire craniomaxillofacial complex: anatomical area of the mouth, jaws, face, skull, as well as associated structures. However, the limited intraoperative visibility, especially the anatomical intricacies, makes this kind of surgery a demanding procedure. Due to the expanding application of computer technology in medicine, computer assisted surgery (CAS) is used increasingly as a supportive tool for the diagnosis, operation planning, and treatment in medicine and dentistry [1-3]. In CAS, the actual intervention is defined as surgical navigation, which has been employed for approximately 20 years, and all use some form of preoperative data, usually in the form of tomographic images combined with some technology to relate these images to the patient. Nowadays, navigation technology has become almost routine in neurosurgery. However, in the field of oral and maxillofacial surgery, computer-aided preoperative planning becomes increasing important and complicated [4, 5], and more complex algorithms in computer graphics and medical image processing are involved.

The purpose of this study is to present an image guided system for oral and maxillofacial surgery, which integrates 3D medical modeling, preoperative surgical planning and intraoperative tracking into a surgical navigation system, named AccuNavi. The framework of the AccuNavi, and various algorithms in the field of computer graphics and medical image processing are discussed in details. With the aid of AccuNavi, surgeons are able to create an exact, detailed plan for the oral and maxillofacial surgery, and then transfer the plan to the operating theatre. A clinical report for a patient with old zygomatic fractures demonstrates the feasibility, reliability and validity of this technology.

II. Material and Methods

The Framework of AccuNavi is described as follows: On the basis of the preoperative data of the CT-scanned patient, image processing (including filter, reformatting, and segmentation) is conducted and 3D-reconstruction of the cranio-maxillofacial structures (including the maxillary sinus and the inferior alveolar nerve) is realized. According to the series of 2D images and the 3D models, preoperative planning is accomplished, including 2D/3D geometrical measurements, bone density analysis, cutting path determination, osteotomy simulation, reposition of the splitted bones, optimization design of the position and orientation of oral implants, bone volume measurement for maxillary defects, simulation of tumor resection and free bone graft, etc. Then, the resulting data of the preoperative planning can be transferred to a self-developed intra-operative navigation system, including the software and hardware. During the surgery, with the support of the optical tracking device of AccuNavi, registration is performed to determine the spatial relationship between Virtual Coordinate System (VCS, refer to as the preoperative image coordinate system) and Real Coordinate Space (RCS, refer to as the patient coordinate system). After registration, there will be constant visualization of the surgical instrument trajectory on the computer screen, while deviation from the preoperative plan position can be detected and displayed in real time, so that the osteotomy procedure can be performed according to the original plan under the guidance of 2D/3D interactive image rendering environment.

The key technology of the software involves some algorithms in the field of medical image processing and computer graphics. The major parts of the algorithms are described as follows:

II.1. DICOM File Parsing

The original import data are usually in DICOM (Digital Imaging in COmmunications and Medicine) format that is widely used to exchange data and provided by various modalities. Gdcm (Grass roots DiCoM), an open-source, C++ library dedicated to reading/parsing and writing Dicom medical files (http://www.creatis.insa-lyon.fr /Public /Gdcm/Main.html), is adopted in this software to handle not only standard but also encapsulated format. Gdcm implements the dicom base standard (part 5) that concentrates on image file format; hence we support the following formats:

- Dicom version 3.0 (including various encodings of JPEG -lossless and lossy-, RLE).
- Papyrus V2 and V3 file headers

II.2. Image Segmentation and 3D- Visualization

A threshold and region growing combined method is adopted so that the object bone tissue, the pixels of which are connected to an initial seed and lie within a lower and upper threshold range, can be segmented out, and then 3D cranio-maxillofacial surface model is reconstructed through the marching cubes algorithm [13] and triangular surface decimation method [14].

II.3. Spline Curve Generation

A spline curve is generated by interpolating a set of coordinate points (i.e., interpolation means that the spline passes through the points). This process is accomplished by adding a sequence of parametric coordinate (t,x) values followed by use of a cardinal basis. Through spline curve generation algorithm, inferior alveolar nerves and a user-defined panoramic curve following the curvature of the jaw bone can be drawn manually.

II.4. Multi-Planar Reconstruction

Multiplanar Reconstruction (MPR) is a post processing technique that reconstructs the axial CT images into panoramic and cross-sectional anatomical planes. Since the orientation of the required cross-sectional images can be specified by the normal of the spline curve at every interpolated coordinate point, it is convenient to extract the slice from the image volume through image interpolation. With respect to panoramic images, at first, every single segmented slice along the spline curve can be extracted from the whole image volume according to the same principle, then; these slices can be merged into one panoramic image.

II.5. Spatial Search and 3D Distance Computing

In order to compute distance between an implant and alveolar nerves (maxillary sinus), an octree-based spatial search algorithm [15] including cell distribution and intersection computing is adopted. Since the 3D models of implants and alveolar nerves (maxillary sinus) are represented in cells (i.e. triangle mesh), the search space is subdivided into smaller parts while octree data structure is defined and the cells can be distributed into buckets of octree. Once the bucket is found, the search is then limited to the cells contained within it. In this way, memory resources and processing time can be greatly reduced.

II.6. Cutting

In order to obtain the sectional image of an implant in 2D views, we need to cut through the 3D model dataset of the implant with a surface (i.e. axial, cross-sectional or panoramic anatomical planes) and then display the interpolated data values on the surface. The cutting algorithm is described as follows: Suppose the implicit function $F(x,y,z)=ax+by+cz-d$ is the cutting surface, then this surface will partition space into 3 areas: $F(x,y,z)<0$, $F(x,y,z)=0$, $F(x,y,z)>0$. For each cell of the 3D model dataset of the implant, function values are generated by evaluating F(x,y,z) for each cell point. If all the points evaluate positive or negative, then the surface does not cut the cell. However, if the points evaluate positive and negative, then the surface passes through the cell[23]. We can use the cell contouring operation to generate the isosurface F(x,y,z)=0 by interpolating along cut edges, which proceeds as follows:

Suppose C1(x0,y0,z0) is the interpolated point for Point A(x1,y1,z1) and Point B(x2,y2,z2), as shown in Figure 2, then the coordinates of C1 can be computed with the following expressions:

$$x_0 = x_1 - \frac{F(x_1, y_1, z_1)}{F(x_2, y_2, z_2) - F(x_1, y_1, z_1)}(x_2 - x_1)$$
$$y_0 = y_1 - \frac{F(x_1, y_1, z_1)}{F(x_2, y_2, z_2) - F(x_1, y_1, z_1)}(y_2 - y_1)$$
$$z_0 = z_1 - \frac{F(x_1, y_1, z_1)}{F(x_2, y_2, z_2) - F(x_1, y_1, z_1)}(z_2 - z_1)$$

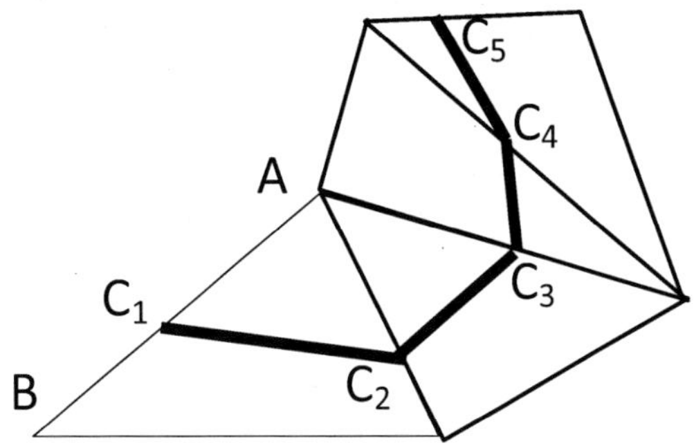

Figure 1. Isosurface generated from cutting.

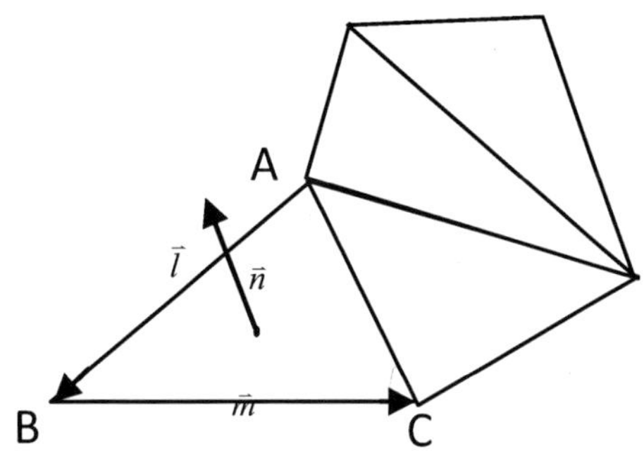

Figure 2. Normal vector of a triangle and measurement for the surface area.

C2, C3, C4, C5, and so on and so forth, can be calculated, and then, the isosurface, i.e. the sectional image, can be generated according to these points (shown in Figure 1).

II.7. Volume Measurement

In order to evaluate bone quality and volume, DTA (Divergence Theorem Algorithm) and MUNC (Maximum Unit Normal Component) method are adopted. Because the 3D reconstructed cranio-maxillofacial models are represented in triangle mesh, the volume measurement expression derived from DTA and MUNC [16, 17] can be simplified as follows:

$$V = k_x \sum_i n_{x_i} c_{x_i} \Delta a_i + k_y \sum_i n_{y_i} c_{y_i} \Delta a_i + k_z \sum_i n_{z_i} c_{z_i} \Delta a_i \quad (1)$$

where k_x represents the number of voxels with maximum unit normal components in the x direction expressed as a fraction of the total number of normals; k_y and k_z are calculated in a similar fashion for the y and z axes; c_{x_i} is the x coordinate of the centroid of the i_{th} triangle, n_{x_i} is the x component of the triangle normal and Δa_i is the triangle area. Suppose the coordinates of the 3 vertex points A,B,C of the i_{th} triangle are respectively (x_1,y_1,z_1), (x_2,y_2,z_2),

(x_3,y_3,z_3), as shown in Figure 2, then the coordinates of the centroid of the triangle can be calculated as follows:

$$c_{x_i} = (x_1 + x_2 + x_3)/3, c_{y_i} = (y_1 + y_2 + y_3)/3, c_{z_i} = (z_1 + z_2 + z_3)/3 \quad (2)$$

The corresponding vectors $\vec{l}, \vec{m}$ of edge $\overrightarrow{AB}, \overrightarrow{BC}$ are:

$$\vec{l} = (x_2 - x_1)\vec{i} + (y_2 - y_1)\vec{j} + (z_2 - z_1)\vec{k} = a_1\vec{i} + b_1\vec{j} + c_1\vec{k} \quad (3)$$

$$\vec{m} = (x_3 - x_2)\vec{i} + (y_3 - y_2)\vec{j} + (z_3 - z_2)\vec{k} = a_2\vec{i} + b_2\vec{j} + c_2\vec{k} \quad (4)$$

Hence, the normal vector

$$\vec{n} = \vec{l} \times \vec{m} = (b_1c_2 - c_1b_2)\vec{i} + (c_1a_2 - a_1c_2)\vec{j} + (a_1b_2 - b_1a_2)\vec{k} \quad (5)$$

So, the x, y, and z components of the normal $\vec{n}$ are:

$$n_{x_i} = (b_1c_2 - c_1b_2)/|\mathrm{\bar{n}}|, n_{y_i} = (c_1a_2 - a_1c_2)/|\mathrm{\bar{n}}|, n_{z_i} = (a_1b_2 - b_1a_2)/|\mathrm{\bar{n}}| \quad (6)$$

where

$$|\mathrm{\bar{n}}| = \sqrt{(b_1c_2 - c_1b_2)^2 + (c_1a_2 - a_1c_2)^2 + (a_1b_2 - b_1a_2)^2} \quad (7)$$

Since the triangle area is calculated as:

$$\Delta a_i = (1/2)\left|\vec{l} \times \vec{m}\right| = (1/2)\left|\vec{n}\right| \quad (8)$$

substitution of equations (2), (6), (7), and (8) into equation (1) leads to the volume of the enclosed surface described by the triangular mesh.

II.8. Registration

The basic requirement of any navigation technique is the registration of the patient's position in relation to the image data set. In this study, ICP (Iterative Closest Point) algorithm [19], an efficient registration method on 3D free-form shapes including point sets, curves, and surfaces, is adopted [18,19]. Suppose the fiducial point sets under the world and virtual coordinate system are respectively P={P_i,i=0,1,2,…,k}, and U={U_i,i=0,1,2,…,n}, where the elements of U and P are not necessary be taken to correspond, as well as the number of them (i.e. k and n) not to be equal, thus, let k≥n.

The computational procedure is described as follows:

1. Compute the closest points: For each point in U, compute the corresponding closest point in P that yields the minimum distance. Let Q denote the resulting set of closest points, $Q=\{q_i, i=0,1,2,\ldots,n\}$.
2. Compute the registration between U and Q via the quaternion–based least squares method so that $\min_{R,T}\sum\|q_i-(Ru_i+T)\|^2$, where R is 3×3 rotation matrix, and T is 3×1 translation matrix.
3. Apply the registration, i.e. let $U_1 = RU + T$.
4. Compute the mean square error between U_1 and Q, and terminate the process if it falls below a preset threshold $\varepsilon>0$ specifying the desired precision of the registration, otherwise, perform the iteration with the substitution of U_1 for U.

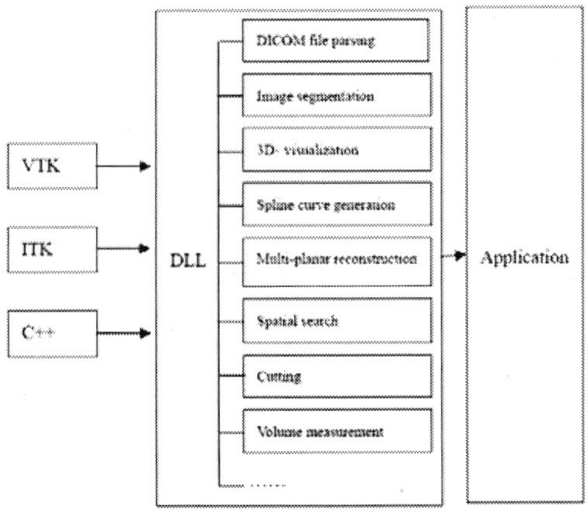

Figure 3. The three-layer modular software model.

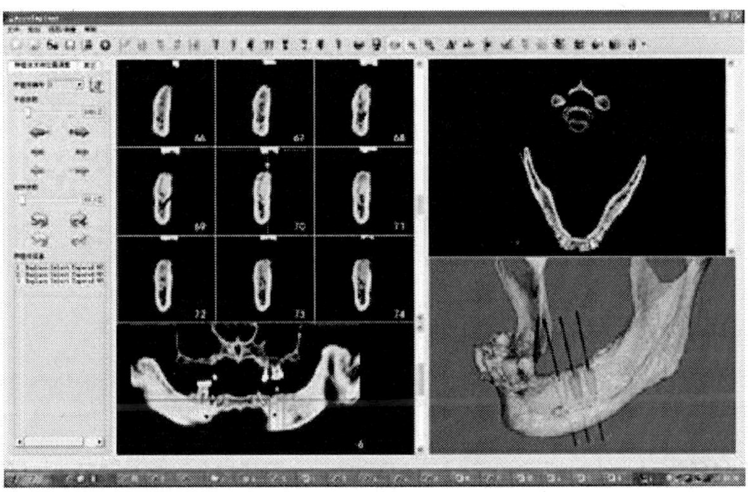

Figure 4. The main interface of the preoperative planning software of AccuNavi.

II.9. Dynamic Link Libraries (DLL)

For each of above-mentioned algorithms, we have developed a set of dynamic link libraries (DLL) using Microsoft Visual C++, as well as the Visualization Toolkit (VTK, an open source, freely available software system for 3D computer graphics, image processing, and visualization etc., http://www.vtk.org/) and Insight Toolkit (ITK, an open-source software toolkit for performing registration and segmentation, http://www.itk.org/) via object oriented programming methodology, therefore, a three-layer modular software model has been developed (shown in Figure 3). This basis can be extended by virtually any new approach or algorithm, which then becomes seamlessly integrated into the method set of the preoperative planning software framework. The aim is to provide well-defined levels of abstraction (the hiding of implementation details) from the individual components, so that new technology can be incorporated into the system without a complete software rewrite. As for graphical user interfaces (GUI), we choose QT (a free, open source, and cross-platform application development framework widely used for the development of GUI programs, http://qt.nokia.com/products) for its powerful cross-platform support features. The main interface of the software is shown in Figure 4.

III. Clinical Applications

The advantage of AccuNavi is validated through clinical applications. In this report, we describe the application of this specialized surgical navigation system for the planning and subsequent precise treatment of old zygomatic fractures (the general information about this patient is listed in Table 1).

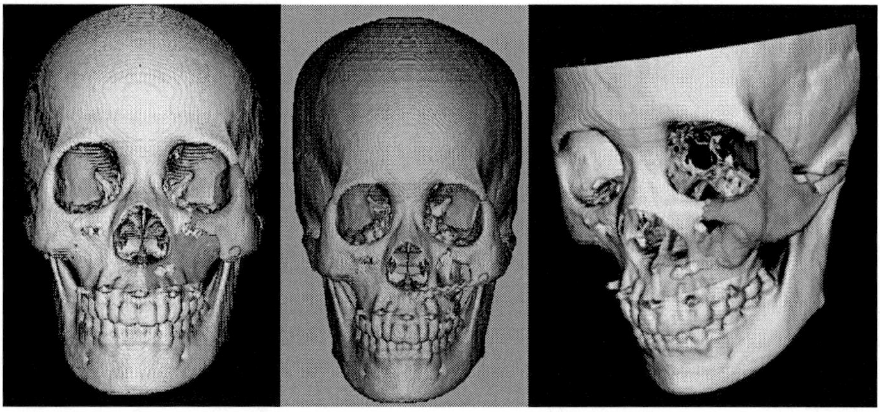

(a) 3D Reconstruction.
(b) The normal parts of the zygoma and maxilla on the right side were mirrored to the left side as benchmark.
(c) The fractured zygoma was then cut and moved to the reference position, and several anatomical landmarks were determined.

Figure 5. Preoperative planning.

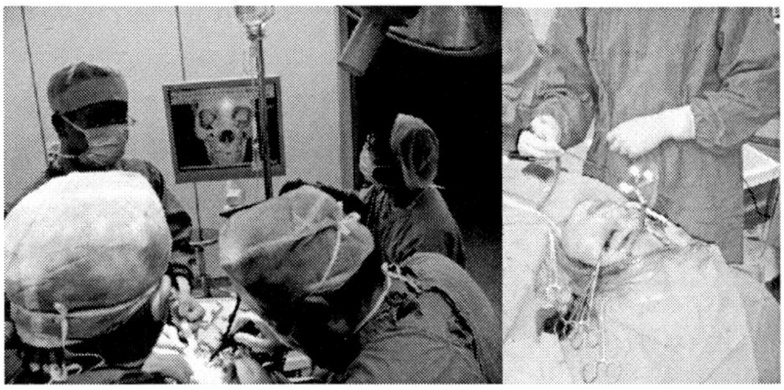

(a) The Cephal-bracket rigidly fixed on the patient's skull bone.
(b) Collecting the coordinates of the fiducial titanium screw markers on the alveolar bone.

Figure 6. Registration procedure.

Table 1. The general information about the patient with old zygomatic fractures

Case	Gender	Age	Diagnosis	Treatment method
1	Female	27	old zygomatic fractures on the left side	The normal parts of the zygoma and maxilla on the right side were mirrored to the left side as benchmark, the fractured zygoma was then cut and moved to the reference position using navigation technology

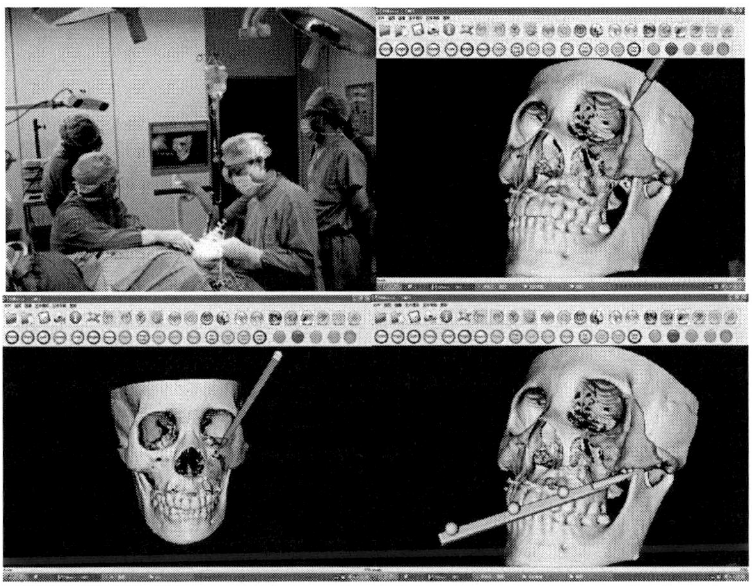

Figure 7. Surgical navigation and screenshot of the software.

First of all, totally 5 titanium screw markers were placed on the patient's alveolar bone as fiducial landmarks for registration. Then, the patient was scanned via a 16-slice spiral CT scanner (GE, LightSpeed, 140KV/250Ma, 0.625mm slice thickenss, 512*512 matrix).The CT data was then imported to AccuNavi for preoperative surgical planning. For this case, according to the discussion of the clinical team, the treatment plan was designed as follows: the crest point, sagittal suture, brow point, anterior nasal spine, etc. were identified to set the mirror plane, then the normal parts of the zygoma and maxilla on the right side were mirrored to the left side as benchmark. After that, the fractured zygoma was then cut and moved to the reference position, and several anatomical landmarks of the fixation region (orbital margin, upper margin of zygomatic arch, etc.) were then determined (shown in Figure 5).

On the day before the surgery, all of the surgical instruments, the rigid bracket assemblies and the retro-reflective balls for tracking, the positioning pointer, etc., were sterilized, and the hardware and software of AccuNavi were both checked to be well-functioned. On the second day, after the patient was in general anaesthesia and the relevant preparative operations were accomplished, the surgeon fixed the Cephal-bracket rigidly on the patient's skull bone. Then, he used a positioning probe to collect the coordinates of the fiducial titanium screw markers on the alveolar bone so that registration was automatically accomplished by AccuNavi (The registration procedure is shown in Figure 6). After registration, there was constant visualization of the cutting trajectory on the computer screen, allowing the surgeon to cut the fractured zygoma according to the original plan under the guidance of AccuNavi. After cutting the fractured zygoma, the surgeon moved it to a proper fixation position. Then, he used the positioning probe to determine whether the fractured bone had been moved to the ideal position according to the preoperative plan. When the tip of the probe was placed on the anatomical landmarks of the fixation region (orbital margin, upper margin of zygomatic arch, etc.), there was constant visualization of the 3D probe model on the computer screen. Then, the surgeon adjusted the position of the fractured bone until the color of the anatomical landmarks turned to red which meant the bone was moved to the position as desired (shown in Figure 7). Finally, the surgeon fixed the fractured bone using titanium plates. The post-operative 3D-reconstructed CT image (shown in Figure 8) demonstrated that the fractured zygoma was fixed in appropriate position and orientation, compared with the preoperative plan.

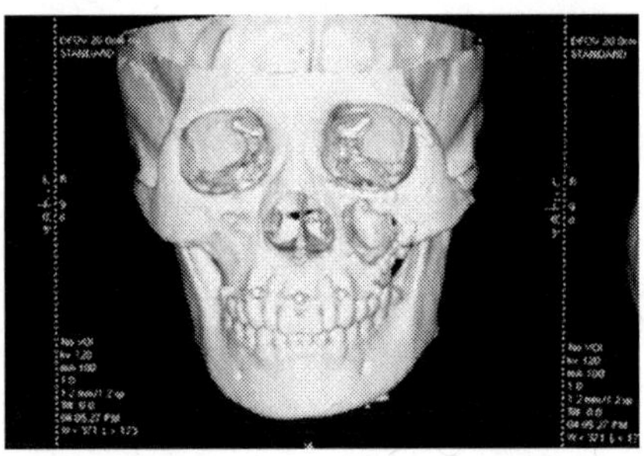

Figure 8. The post-operative 3D-reconstructed CT image.

IV. Discussion and Conclusion

Computer-assisted oral and maxillofacial surgery is the modern surgical approach in orthognathic surgery (correction of the anomalies of the jaws and skull), in temporomandibular joint (TMJ) surgery, or in the reconstruction of the mid-face and orbit, etc. [1-12] However, the planning of complex surgical procedures necessitates highly reliable algorithms in computer graphics and medical image processing. Various algorithms are explicitly discussed, and a plug-in evolutive software architecture is introduced in this study. By separating the software into several DLL divisions, we enhance modularity and flexibility in our system. It is really more accessible than rewriting the entire software in terms of adding new functionalities, including image processing algorithms, graphical user interface, data management components, etc. Other advantages of using DLLs include reduced code footprint, lower memory utilization due to single-copy-sharing, flexible development and testing, and functional isolation. Since the current operating systems for the software is only based on Windows, our future work is to develop a cross-platform (Windows, Linux and Mac Os X operating systems) application environment. With the introduction of DLL, this task can be easily accomplished since the only platform-dependent part of the library is the graphical user interface. Nevertheless, a clinical report for a patient with old zygomatic fractures reveals that AccuNavi is very helpful in oral and maxillofacial surgery. However, more clinical cases will be done to demonstrate its feasibility and reliability.

ACKNOWLEDGMENT

This study was supported by Natural Science Foundation of China (Grant No.:51005156).The authors would also like to thank Ms. Catherine Liu for reviewing the manuscripts and offering constructive criticisms, which were incorporated in the final form.

REFERENCES

[1] Zachow, S; Hege, HC; Deuflhard, P. Computer Assisted Planning in Cranio-Maxillofacial Surgery. *Journal of Computing and Information Technology-Special Issue on Computer-Based Craniofacial Modelling and Reconstruction*, 2006, 14(1), 53-64.

[2] Chabanas, M; Payan, Y. Finite element model of the face soft tissue for computer-assisted maxillofacial surgery, *proceedings of the Fifth International Symposium on Computer Methods in Biomechanics and Biomedical Engineering*, CMBBE'2001, Rome, Italy, November 2001.

[3] Hassfeld, S; Muhling, J. Computer assisted oral and maxillofacial surgery – a review and an assessment of technology. *International Journal of Oral Maxillofacial Surgery*, 2001, 30(1), 2-13.

[4] Troulis, MJ; Everett, P; Seldin, EB; Kikinis, R; Kaban, LB. Three-dimensional treatment planning system based on computed tomographic data. *International Journal of Oral Maxillofacial Surgery*, 2002, 31(4), 349-357.

[5] James, Xia; Nabil Samman, Richie, WK. Yeung, Dongfeng Wang, Steve G.F. Shen, Horace H.S. Ip, Henk Tideman. Computer-assisted three-dimensional surgical planning and simulation 3D soft tissue planning and prediction. *International Journal of Oral and Maxillofacial Surgery*, 2000, 29(4), 250-258.

[6] Ming-Dar Tsai, Ming-Shium Hsieh, Shyan-Bin Jou. Virtual reality orthopedic surgery simulator. *Computers in Biology and Medicine*, 2001, 31(5), 333-351.

[7] James Mah, Reyes Enciso. The Virtual Craniofacial Patient-A Platform for the Future of Craniofacial Healthcare. *The 29th Annual Moyers Symposium*, 2002.

[8] Westermark, A; Zachow, S; Eppley, B. 3-D osteotomy planning in maxillofacial surgery, including soft tissue prediction. *Journal of Craniofacial Surgery*, 2005, 16(1), 100-104.

[9] Ayoub, AF; Xiao, Y; Khambay, B; Siebert, JP; Hadley, D. Towards. Building a photo-realistic virtual human face for craniomaxillofacial diagnosis and treatment planning. *International Journal of Oral and Maxillofacial Surgery*, 2007, 36(5), 423-428.

[10] http://www.zib.de/visual/projects/cas/caslong.en.html

[11] *http://www.materialise.com/materialise/view/en/92530-SurgiCase* + CMF.html

[12] http://www.medicim.com/products_maxilim.html

[13] Lorensen, WE; Cline, HE. Marching cubes: A high resolution 3D surface construction algorithm. *ACM Computer Graphics*, 1987, 21, 38-44.

[14] Schroeder, WJ; Zarge, JA; Lorensen, WE. Decimation of triangle meshes. *Proceedings ACMM Siggraph*, 1992, 26, 65-70.

[15] Schroeder, W; Martin, K; Lorensen, B. The Visualization Toolkit: *An Object-Oriented Approach To 3D Graphics*, Prentice Hall, 1997.

[16] Lancaster, JL; Eberly, D; Alyassin, A; Hunter, DJ; Fox, PT. A geometric model for measurement of surface distance, surface area, and volume from tomographic images. *Med. Phys.*, 1992, 19, 419-431.

[17] Hughes, SW; D'Arcy, TJ; Maxwell, DJ; Saunders, JE; Ruff, CF; Chiu, WS; Sheppard, RJ. Application of a new discreet form of Gauss' theorem for measuring volume. *Phys. Med. Biol.*, 1996, 41, 1809-1821.

[18] Arun, KS; Huang, TS; Blostein, SD. Least-squares fitting of two 3-D point sets. IEEE Trans. *Pattern Anal. Mach. Intell.*, 1987, 9, 698-700.

[19] Besl, PJ; Mckay, ND. A method for Registration of 3D shapes. IEEE Trans. *Pattern Anal. Mach. Intell.*, 1992, 14, 239-256.

In: Computer Graphics
Editor: Martin J. Davis

ISBN: 978-1-61761-811-6

Chapter 4

IMPROVEMENT PROPOSAL IN THE TREATMENT AND DISSEMINATION OF THE RESULTS OF COMPUTER GRAPHICS IN THE STUDY AND ANALYSIS OF CULTURAL HERITAGE

José Ignacio Rojas-Sola[1*], Miguel Castro-García[1] and María del Pilar Carranza-Cañada[2]

[1]University of Jaén, Department of Engineering Graphics, Design and Projects, Campus de las Lagunillas, Jaén 23071, Spain

[2]University of Córdoba, Campus de Rabanales, Department of Engineering Graphics and Geomatics, Córdoba 14071, Spain

ABSTRACT

The diverse nature of the term COMPUTER GRAPHICS can be seen in the high number of keywords associated with it. This paper deals with a topic of increasing relevance, that of the use of computer graphics applications in the process of valuing cultural heritage: identification, records and research, protection, training, conservation and restoration, value and dissemination, management of heritage and new technologies.

Research in the field of cultural heritage has benefited from the evolution of the technology of computer graphics, which has undergone exponential development over the last decades. Today it is possible to undertake research which without the aid of modern computers would imply enormous mathematical effort, or which would simply not be possible.

Some of the examples which can be stated are the ability to obtain *in situ* exact virtual models (VM) of heritage elements, their representation and geo-referenced analysis using Geographical Information Systems (GIS), the techniques of Augmented Reality (AR) in the virtual recreations of cultural sites, or the advanced structural analyses which increase our understanding of techniques in use in ancient times.

---

[*] Corresponding author. Professor José Ignacio Rojas-Sola, PhD. University of Jaén, Department of Engineering Graphics, Design and Projects, Campus de las Lagunillas, Jaén 23071. Spain. Tel: +34-953-212452; Fax: +34-953-212334; Email: jirojas@ujaen.es

As a result, there is much excellent research which studies this cultural heritage, although in many cases the dissemination of the results is partial, and therefore does not fully exploit the educational facet of the research. For example, this is often published in the form of articles, and the multimedia information which is fundamental is lost.

This paper attempts to show how a Learning Management System (LMS) has been used in the recuperation of an example of Industrial Heritage, the *San Francisco* windmill (Véjer de la Frontera, Cádiz, Spain). An open source Content Management System (CMS) is chosen to house the results of the use of Computer Graphics in the field of engineering graphics.

Introduction

Archaeology is area with a broad span of knowledge. Any aspect of ancient societies is studied through original material remains, using diverse prospection and analysis techniques. Although many there are many different archaeological disciplines, this chapter deals with studies and analyses undertaken in the field of industrial archaeology.

Archaeological studies in industrial fields are supported using other scientific areas, with the aim, during the analysis stage, of obtaining a single reality from different viewpoints, which generate results of different natures leading to more accurate and complete conclusions.

One of the scientific areas used both in analysis of and in recording data in this field is computer-aided design (CAD). This is a tool which can represent an archaeological reality under study using models which allow viewing of the elements studied and which later serve as a basis for historical, social or mechanical analyses, amongst others. Thanks to info-realistic graphical representation, it is possible to show the different states of any material example of cultural heritage, allowing for research into the events and processes which have taken place over time.

CAD techniques allow the generation of two- and three-dimensional models which form the basis of study for other scientific disciplines. It is possible to carry out studies of virtual physical or chemical processes which simulate the degradation of and variations in the intrinsic properties of a material, as well as mechanical studies, such as a tension analysis using the Finite Elements Method (FEM) or a surface study using a curvature analysis. This shows the enormous potential which graphical computing offers to archaeological studies.

The aim of this chapter is to tackle the process of dissemination of the results produced in a study on cultural heritage, with appropriate use of graphical information applied to a study of industrial archaeology. The study deals with the cultural heritage of the windmills of Andalusia (Spain). The possibility exists to generate Learning Objects (LOs), a tool for training students and future researchers in the area, as is the case in other disciplines [1].

To this end, first, the possibility is analyzed of generating LOs which are specific to graphic engineering in industrial archaeology. Once the educational resources are known, that should be described using metadata which meet a standard and a series of stipulated requirements. The result is a specific vocabulary to define metadata pertaining to Computer Graphics in a standard and concise manner. This allows access, management and re-use of LO resources via E-learning platforms.

Graphical Representation in Industrial Archaelogy

Computer Graphics provides two principal functions to industrial archaeology.

The first function deals with solving the problem of recording graphically the different archaeological elements which make up any example of industrial heritage. The representation of reality is initially made in two dimensions, and the information used stems from archaeological prospection and other related studies, such as historical or geographical studies. All the information is contained in general and detailed plans, and can be reconstructed if the object represented were to be lost.

CAD techniques provide the possibility to store and study this information, which is usually represented on plans, and this type of graphical record is present during the initial stages of work in industrial archaeology. However, it is common to represent all the material elements three-dimensionally, where the degree of detail achieved depends on the result which is sought and the recording technique used. Once the objects have been modeled in 3D, it is possible, from the information obtained from archaeological digs or from previous research, to represent the scene from an info-realist perspective. The techniques used for this task are material texturing, natural illumination and computer animation, both of the moving parts of objects and of other types of auxiliary elements, such as particles or effects of physics or the environment, among others. The exit format of this type of representation is usually a bitmap or a video clip. Figure 1 shows a bitmap from a study of the recovery of a windmill which forms part of the cultural heritage of Andalusia (Spain).

The second function is the development of 3D models of archaeological remains, which would form the starting point for various scientific disciplines. It is therefore necessary for the model to be as true to life as possible, so that in the analysis stage accurate results can be obtained. This is the reason why 3D laser scanners are an ideal solution in order to achieve this aim. One example of this type of analysis is shown in Figure 2, which represents a curvature analysis using a Gaussian model of the end of the main axle of the windmill under study.

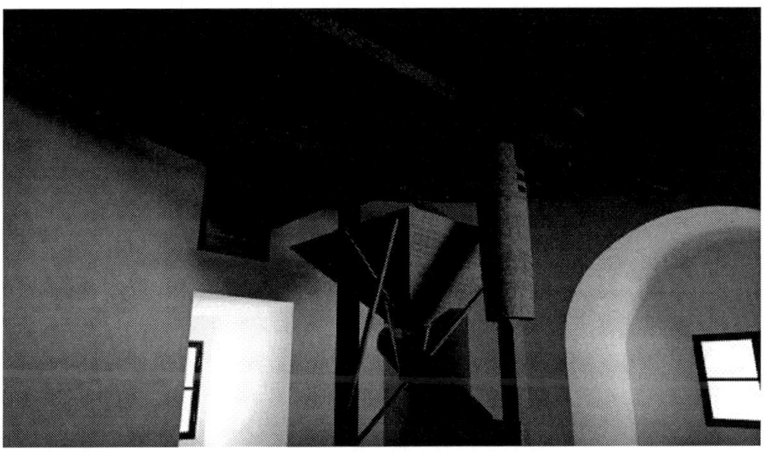

Figure 1. Bitmap of the graphical information of the San Francisco windmill (Véjer de la Frontera, Cádiz, Spain).

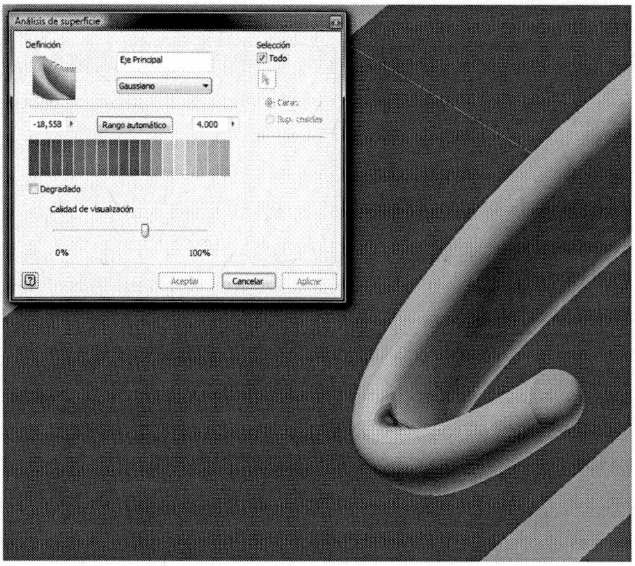

Figure 2. Curvature analysis of the 3D model of the windmill axle.

Analysis of the Learning Objects

Once the potential and the main resources provided by computer graphics for industrial archaeology have been shown, the next step is the extraction of metadata (data which contain information about the data themselves) which can describe the LOs arising from this scientific discipline.

Based on the two types of resources provided by computer graphics analyzed above, the principal LOs are related to the generation of plans or 3D models and the creation of multimedia results with different degrees of info-realism. Therefore, there are three large sets which cover the most important stages in learning in this discipline: Projection Systems, Modeling Techniques and Rendering.

Projection Systems

Projection systems belong to the field of descriptive geometry, the aim of which is to represent bodies using projections such which can be converted from 2D to 3D and vice versa. The importance of choosing one representation system or another lies in the geometric operations which have to be undertaken to change dimensions and the intention of the representation.

Therefore, one of the key indicators for classifying LOs is the type of projection system used to obtain the results of the research in plan form. The representation systems (Figure 3) most widely used for these plans are:

- Orthographic projection: a parallel and orthogonal projection system with two perpendicular projection planes. It allows measurements to be taken and is used for 2D representations.

- Contour map: a parallel and orthogonal projection system with a single projection plane. It allows measurements to be taken and is used for 2D representations.
- Axonometric system: a projection system which is parallel and orthogonal to a tri-rectangular trihedron, and orthogonal or oblique to a single plane, according to its axonometry. It is used for 3D perspective representations.

Modeling Techniques

The CAD modeling process consists of creating graphical representations using software which provides 2D or 3D records of the information taken from archaeological digs or from reference bibliography. The choice of the modeling technique depends in each study on the type of object or on the subsequent processing. Specifically, in the field of windmills, it is necessary to consider that the 3D model can be completed in part or totally by the use of three different modeling techniques (Figure 4): solid modeling, surface modeling and generative modeling.

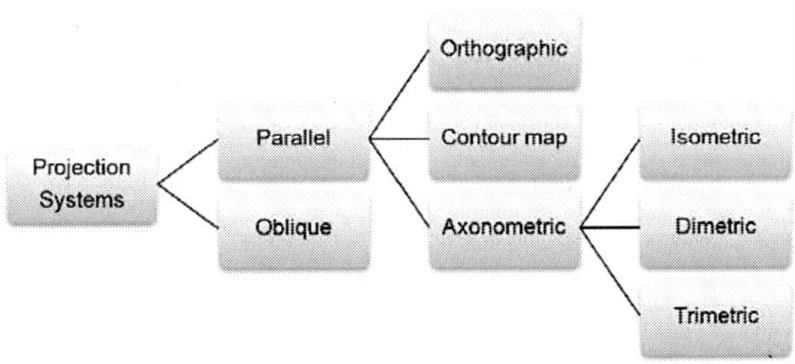

Figure 3. Main projection systems.

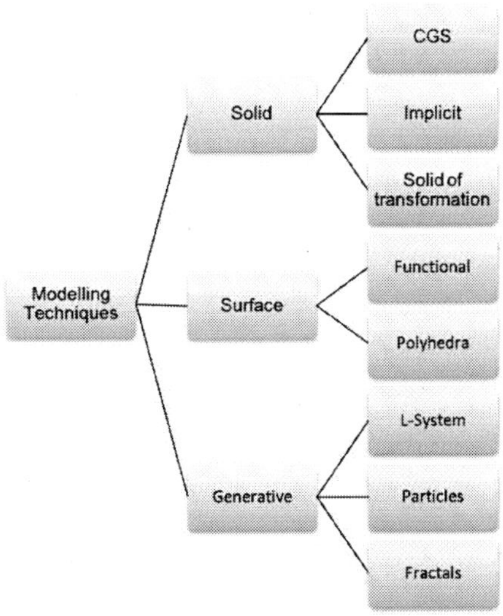

Figure 4. Main modeling techniques.

In solid modeling 3D models are obtained using constructive solid geometry (CSG) techniques, either implicitly or using transformation solids, which can respond to inherent physical or chemical characteristics.

Surface modeling consists of a technique in which the 3D models obtained are created using meshes which can of different types, such as polygonal, NURBS or T-Spline, among others. This technique is widely used in many simulation and animation programs, and is very useful in studying different aspects such as FEM, curvature analysis or thermodynamics, among others.

Generative modeling covers a range of techniques which are based on natural directives, adjusting the most appropriate technique to given solids. These techniques can be roughly classified into L-System (also known as Lidenmayer), particles and fractals.

Rendering

The final key stage in the educational process in the field of Computer Graphics applied to industrial heritage is the rendering of 3D models. The rendering process is gives a raster graphics image which contains information about the texture and lighting, giving exit formats which are appropriate for multimedia. Thus, results are obtained with a degree of realism which depends on the needs of the work undertaken. In general, four types of rendering are used (Figure 5).

Radiosity

This is the first method which was used to simulate the interaction of light beams in their intersection with a surface. This technique allows the creation of more realistic scenes using more elaborate shading, taking the properties of color and type of reflection from the surface itself. In this way, nearby objects are influenced by the objects rendered.

Scanline Rendering

This second type of rendering uses an algorithm to determine the visible surface in a 3D scene. It works on a row-by-row basis, in which the polygons are presented in order of their coordinates. The algorithm has variations, such as Z-buffer, in order to improve its performance.

Ray casting

Ray casting uses the algorithm of the same name that was presented by Arthur Appel in 1968 [2]. The rendering process is carried out using light rays which are cast from the perspective of the observer. One of the limits of this method is that it does not consider the effects produced by the light rebounding off other objects, which makes it impossible to create reflections and refractions, which means that the final result has a lesser degree of realism.

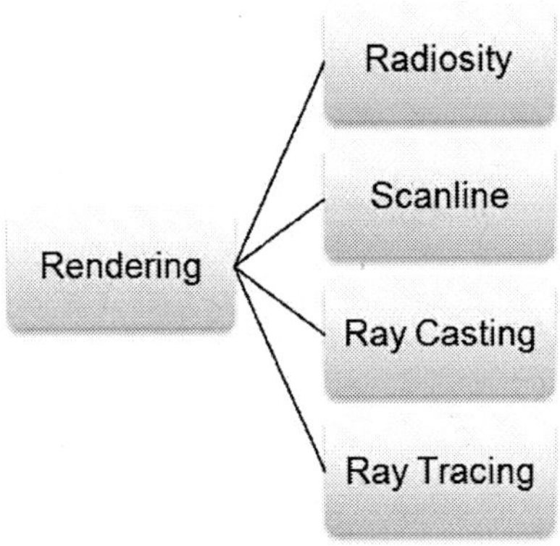

Figure 5. Main rendering techniques.

Ray Tracing

This last type of rendering is considered to be the most complete, as the process of calculation takes into account the three new light rays from the interaction of the incident ray with the work surface. Thus, the effects of refraction, reflection and shadow are modeled.

STRUCTURING OF LEARNING OBJECTS

Recent technologies applied to the field of education make up a set of applications which have shown that communication between them and the resources used, such as LOs, should conform to a set of standards. Thus the knowledge database for E-learning has a wide dimension, while being widely accessible, irrespective of country, language or any other aspect.

Therefore, given the importance of computer graphics in the field of industrial engineering, and having analyzed the three important keys for obtaining LOs from the research, the next step is to select and apply the current standards which regulate the creation of the metadata necessary for the LOs.

Today, the most important organizations which set out standards for E-learning platforms are Interoperable Learning Technology (IMS), Aviation Industry CBT (AICC), Alliance of Remote Authoring and Distribution Networks (ARIADNE) and Advance Distributed Learning (ADL). In addition, there are organizations which develop integrated standards such as ISO, IEEE or CEN/ISSS.

The specification which is analyzed in this chapter is the Sharable Content Object Reference Model (SCORM), specifically the SCORM 2004 3rd Edition. This is a standard which aims to become the final and unique model for creating metadata of the educational resources which are used in E-learning platforms. This standard has been developed by ADL, while considering the work of other institutions in the standardization of metadata, such as IEEE, IMS and EML (the latter from the Open University of the Netherlands, OUNL). In addition, the idea of ADL was to obtain four high level requirements in its standard: reusability, accessibility, durability and interoperability. SCORM is structured in three technical areas:

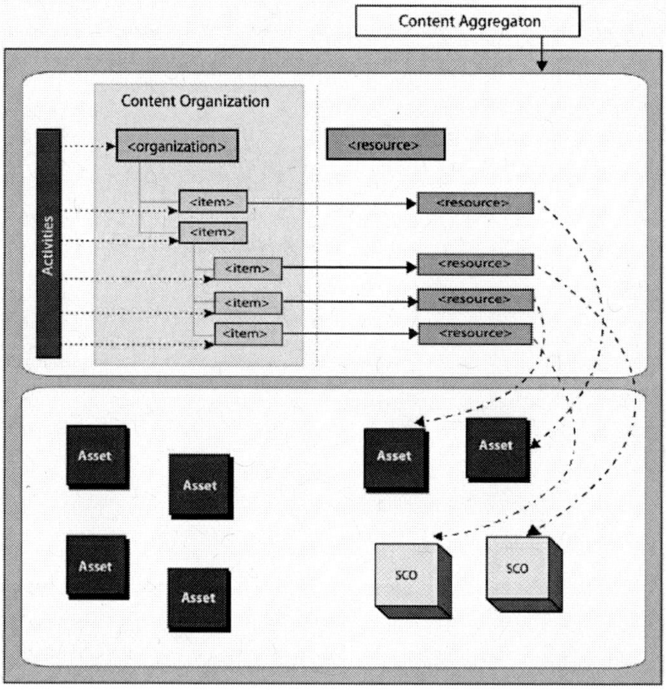

Figure 6. Conceptual Illustration of a Content Aggregation Model [4].

- Content Aggregation Model (CAM): this is centered on the description of the components which make up learning as well as those of the package. This means that these components are interchangeable between different platforms, along with the structuring of the information which is used to identify them.
- Run-Time Environment (RTE): this book deals with the interoperability between Sharable Content Objects (SCOs) and Learning Management Systems (LMSs) or Learning Content Management Systems (LCMSs).
- Sequencing and Navigation (SN): This last book offers relative information in the operation processes of sequencing and navigation which are carried out by LMSs.

The modeling of SCORM content covers the different elements which make up SCORM CAM, and the educational resources are appropriate to an e-learning system. The concept map of a CAM structure is shown in Figure 6 [3].

The Asset is the most basic element among learning resources. It can be made up of data in various formats, such as mp3 audio, XML documents, jpeg, Flash objects or JavaScript functions, among others. However, there is a higher level formed by the Asset, whose main characteristic is that it can communicate with a LMS or LMCS using the standard proposed by IEEE; this type of element is known as SCO.

The Activities are made up of the framework which should be generated by the person responsible for creating resources or a learning environment, such as the content of a course or an exercise in self-learning. This framework leads to an organization of content with a vertical hierarchy, using subactivities. These subactivities can be associated with educational resources such as Asset or SCO.

Once the SCORM Content Model Components have been established, it is necessary to find the way in which the educator can obtain the information from all its elements. This can be done thanks to the metadata which provide information about the data themselves. To this end SCORM is based on the IEEE standard 1484.12.1-2002 Learning Object Metadata (LOM) [5]. In addition, there is no defined SCORM directive to describe SCORM Content Model Components, and so it is necessary to use IEEE LOM.

LOM XML Schema Definition [3, 6] has 64 metadata elements, of which SCORM classifies as "Mandatory" those which must be taken into account. The other elements are considered as "Optional" or "Not Permitted" according to their classification. The metadata in SCORM have the parent instance <lom> on which depend the child instances; of these, the mandatory elements are: <general>, <lifeCycle>, <metaMetadata>, <technical>, <educa-ional>, <rights>, <relation>, <annotation> y <classification>. Each child has specific-ations or relationships with other elements [7] and can have vocabulary tokens which have previously been defined and are globally accepted.

However, the aim of this chapter is to define specific vocabulary for the metadata of the different educational resources which can be taken from Computer Graphics, in the field of industrial archaeology. Therefore, specific vocabulary is created for the child <classification> which fulfils the requirements of best practice according to the specifications of LOM XML Binding [8].

```
<imsmd:lom>
  <imsmd:classification>
    <imsmd:purpose>
      <imsmd:source>COMPUTER GRAPHICS v1.0</imsmd:source>
      <imsmd:value>discipline</imsmd:value>
    </imsmd:purpose>
  </imsmd:classification>
</imsmd:lom>
```

Figure 7. Code example of <purpose> element

<purpose>

This element describes the purpose which will make a general classification of the CAM. IEEE LOM defines <source> as a subelement of <purpose>. The value of this parameter in specific vocabulary is considered as "COMPUTER GRAPHICS v1.0". The subelement <value> has its own vocabulary tokens, and in this case "discipline" is selected from the possible options (Figure 7).

<taxonPath>

The objective of <taxonPath> is to describe a specific classification system using a correct taxonomic path. This element is divided into two child elements: <source> and <taxon>.

<source> is used to describe or name the chosen classification system. The name of the proposed classification system is: "GC1.0" which stands for "COMPUTER GRAPHICS v1.0".

<taxon> is used to refer to a specific field within a taxonomy, and is the node which defines a label or term of the system itself. It has an alphanumeric structure and has two child elements: <id> and <entry>. These can be used simultaneously or it is possible that only one of the two is needed. In the formulation of specific vocabulary the child <id> has been chosen as obligatory, as it is sufficient to define the specific term of the taxonomy. Figures 8, 9 and 10 show the different <id> educational resources mentioned above.

Figure 11 shows a fragment of code in which the "CM1" label has been selected, which refers to the educational resource: Projection System → Parallel → Contour Maps.

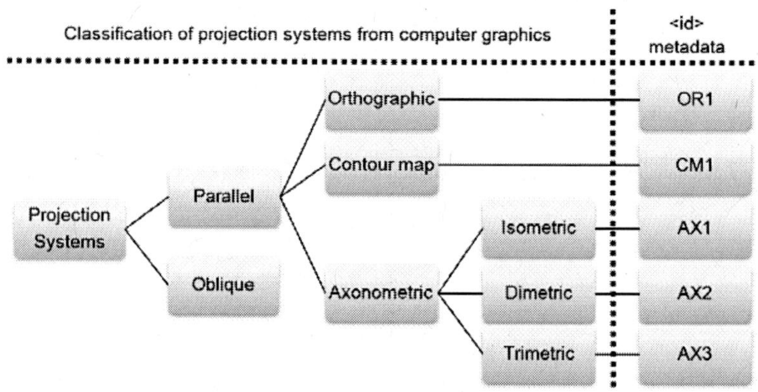

Figure 8. Classification of projection systems from computer graphics.

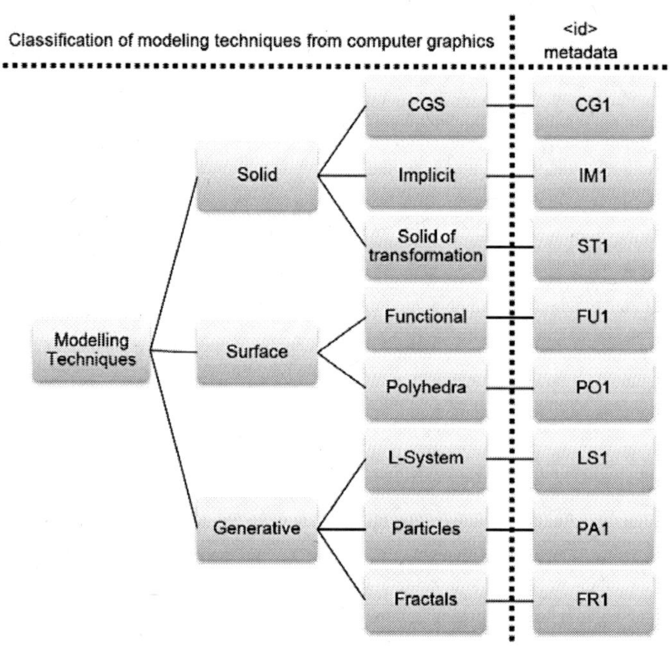

Figure 9. Classification of modeling techniques from computer graphics.

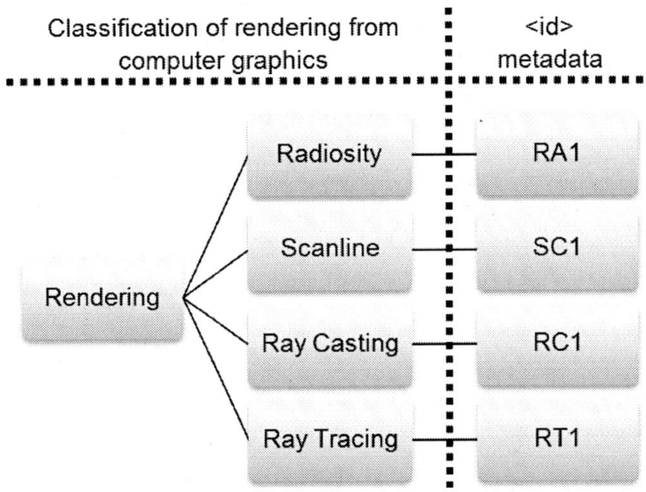

Figure 10. Classification of rendering from computer graphics.

```
<imsmd:lom>
 <imsmd:classification>
  <imsmd:taxonPath>
     <imsmd:source>
       <imsmd:string>CG1.0</imsmd:string>
     </imsmd:source>
     <imsmd:taxon>
       <imsmd:id>CM1</imsmd:id>
     </imsmd:taxon>
   </imsmd:taxonPath>
 </imsmd:classification>
</imsmd:lom>
```

Figure 11. Code example of <taxonPath> element.

<description>

<description> creates an idea of the purpose, in this case the discipline, using a structured explanation in LangString data format. In the proposed vocabulary system, this element is "Optional", and is used if it is necessary to develop an idea which is not fully expressed in the <keyword> element. Figure 12 shows an example of <description> about the resource "CM1".

```
<imsmd:lom>
  <imsmd:classification>
    <imsmd:description>
      <imsmd:string>The system whereby maps are generated with parallel projection</imsmd:string>
    </imsmd:description>
  </imsmd:classification>
</imsmd:lom>
```

Figure 12. Code example of <description> element.

<keyword>

Lastly, this element covers the keywords which describe in detail the purpose, which in this case is "discipline". Figure 13 shows a code example of the keywords which correspond to the elements <purpose> and <id>.

```
<imsmd:lom>
  <imsmd:classification>
    <imsmd:keyword>
      <imsmd:string>projection system parallel contour maps</imsmd:string>
    </imsmd:keyword>
  </imsmd:classification>
</imsmd:lom>
```

Figure 13. Code example of <keyword> element.

CONCLUSION

It has been shown that Computer Graphics is a broad discipline which is used as a tool in other areas such as industrial archaeology, showing its usefulness in the recovery of cultural heritage.

The graphic work of this research has shown three large sets of educational resources: Projection Systems, Modeling Techniques and Rendering, which can generate LOs; these in turn are described using metadata formulated with the development of specific vocabulary in the discipline of Computer Graphics. This means that they can be easily located and reused by educators who are specialized in e-learning platforms, such as LMS and LCMS

FUNDING

This research has been developed thanks to the Excellence Research Project sponsored by the Department of Innovation, Science and Enterprise of Andalusian Regional Government (Spain), entitled "*Historical Heritage of Andalusia windmills*".

REFERENCES

[1] Latorre, M., Díaz, G., Castro, M., Sancristóbal, E., García, F. & Piere, J. (2008). Diseño de un Entorno de Simulación Eléctrica basado en Objetos de Aprendizaje. *X International Symposium on Computers in Education* (SIIE 2008), 323-328.

[2] Appel, A. (1968). Some techniques for machine rendering of solids. *AFIPS Conference Proc.*, *32*, 37-45.

[3] LOM XML Schema Definition. Available from: *http://ltsc.ieee.org/xsd/lomv1.0*

[4] Paul, J. (2009). SCORM® 2004 4th Edition Content Aggregation Model (CAM) Version 1.1. Available at: *http :// www. adlnet. gov /Pages/ Default.aspx*

[5] IEEE, (2005). IEEE 1484.12.1-2002 Learning Object Metadata Standard. *Institute of Electrical and Electronics Engineers*. Available at: *http://www.ieee.org*

[6] W3C, (2006). Extensible Markup Language (XML) 1.1 (Second Edition). Available at: *http://www.w3.org/TR/xml11*

[7] Lu, E. J., Horng, G., Yu, C. & Chou L. (2010). Extended Relation Metadata for SCORM-based Learning Content Management Systems. *Educational Technology & Society*, *13*, 220-235.

[8] Carnegie Mellon University, (2003). Best Practices Guide for Content Developers 1st Ed. Pittsburgh: *Learning Systems Architecture Lab*.

In: Computer Graphics
Editor: Martin J. Davis

ISBN: 978-1-61761-811-6

Chapter 5

OPEN-SOURCE AND FREEWARE TOOLS FOR COMPUTER GRAPHICS

***Andrés Iglesias*[*] *and Akemi Gálvez*[†]**
Department of Applied Mathematics and Computational Sciences,
University of Cantabria, E.T.S.I. Caminos, Canales y Puertos,
Avda. de los Castros, s/n, E-39005, Santander, Spain

Abstract

The emergence of freeware and open-source software has been unanimously regarded as a technological breakthrough in recent years. Many freeware programs and packages are now widely used by individuals and corporations. Simultaneously, open-source codes are being increasingly incorporated into powerful (not only free but also proprietary) systems and applications. This process is also apparent in computer graphics, where freeware and open-source software is now getting outstanding levels of social and technological acceptance among professional users and companies. In this chapter we explore the on-going changes currently happening within the computer graphics community as a consequence of this process. In particular, the chapter discusses some issues related to this new approach, such as the kind of licenses available and their implications for further use. We also provide pointers to a large collection of open-source and freeware tools and middleware available to handle just about every development task, briefly emphasizing their potential advantages and drawbacks with respect to their proprietary counterparts. Open-source and freeware tools are described and classified in order to provide our readers with a repository of websites and links where freely-available software can be smoothly downloaded and installed. Some hints to help our readers to use the appropriate software for specific tasks are also reported.

Keywords: Computer graphics, video games, rendering engine, open-source, freeware, GPL, LGPL, copyleft, computer modeling.

AMS Subject Classification: 65D17, 65D18, 68N15, 68U05, 68U07, 68U20, 68U35.

[*]E-mail address: iglesias@unican.es; Web site: http://personales.unican.es/ iglesias
[†]E-mail address: galveza@unican.es

1. Introduction

Traditionally, Computer Graphics has been primarily regarded as a budget-first field. At the dawning age of computers, its use was limited to a restricted club of universities and research labs, where a few visionaries saw the possibilities of computers as a valuable resource for yielding graphical output. At that time, computer graphics was an elitist - and often marginal - activity with not apparent influence in common people's life. However, the work of those pioneers make it possible the advent of personal computers and arcade games that popularized computer graphics all over the world during the 70s and 80s. Digital images and videogames become ubiquitous and new exciting developments appeared in several fields such as entertainment and movies industries, design and manufacturing, advertisement and many others. The invention of microchip (or integrated circuit) and its great development spurred the production of minicomputers and microcomputers, which were small and inexpensive enough for small businesses and even schools to own. The microchip also led to the microprocessor, another important breakthrough technology in the development of the personal computer. As a result, computers moved from a small market of hundreds of extremely expensive units to a huge mass production for individual users. Those end-users benefited greatly from the fact that hardware prices decreased in the 70s and 80s, and software became more adaptable. Increased innovation (famously summarized by Moore's Law), high volume production and intense competition among hardware suppliers paved the way for the amazing level of computer penetration we enjoy in today's technological world.

But while new generations of avid high-tech consumers put their eyes on computer graphics and digital media, there was a insurmountable gap between computer graphics users and creators. Even when software and hardware costs started to decline and computer equipment became affordable for general public, especialized graphical cards and expensive proprietary software prevented individual users from creating their own digital visual content. Computer movies and videogames were the realm of large companies where task force is typically measured in terms of thousands of person/month and budgets account for millions of dollars for any single project. Even the medium-sized companies and corporations experienced serious difficulties to access to a market where the outcomes quality was so linked to the huge sum of prohibitive hardware equipment, expensive software tools, skilled technical staff and substantial time required to bring a professional computer graphics project to life. Fortunately, this discouraging scenario have changed dramatically during the last few years. A nice combination of affordable hardware resources and a wealth of open-source and freeware tools are now available to companies and end-users in order to yield high-quality graphical output. In this chapter we explore this on-going democratization process currently happening within the computer graphics community as a results of those changes. In particular, the chapter discusses some issues related to this new approach, such as the kind of licenses available and their implications for further use. We also provide pointers to a large collection of open-source and freeware tools and middleware available to handle just about every development task, emphasizing their potential advantages and drawbacks with respect to their proprietary counterparts. Open-source and freeware tools are described and classified in order to provide our readers with a repository of websites and links where freely-available software can be smoothly downloaded and installed. Some hints to help our readers to use the appropriate software for specific tasks are also reported.

Potential audience for this chapter is virtually any person interested in computer graphics, computer animation and videogames, with emphasis upon code developers, software managers, computer science students and teachers, small and medium sized computer graphics software companies, free-lance developers and end-users. We should remark however that the chapter has been influenced by both the huge magnitude of this task and the limitations of space. Some references have had to be omitted and many explanations have been reduced to the minimum. Due to these reasons, neither the description nor the bibliographic entries in this chapter are intended to comprise a totally exhaustive survey on the subject. However, we hope that we have included enough comments and references to make the chapter useful to our readers.

2. Understanding License Issues

Although usually computer graphics is mostly about computer modeling and animation, software development and so on, it is always convenient to take a look at the legal issues of what you are going to do. Before throwing yourself into your computer graphics project, take a break, breath deeply and read the EULA (short for *End-User License Agreement*, also referred to as the *software license* or *user license*), the most common type of license for software. An EULA is a legal contract between the manufacturer and/or the author and the end-user of an application. In general, it details how the software can and cannot be used and any restrictions that the manufacturer imposes (for instance, most EULAs of proprietary software prohibit the user from sharing the software with anyone else, performing reverse engineering to get the source code of the software or modifying it in case it is available). As in typical legal contracts, the EULA protects both parties from liability if the software is used in a way not intended by the manufacturer or author.

Of course, the user has the option of not accepting the EULA, subsequently surrendering the rights and ability to use the software. And there are many different ways to do it: some contracts stipulate acceptance of the agreement simply by opening the shrink-wrapped package; some others require the user to mail back to the manufacturer a signed agreement; some others ask the user to accept the agreement after the application is installed by clicking on an acceptance form that appears on users monitor (such as the applications downloaded from the Internet). Finally, and this is the most important thing here: whether or not you accept EULA conditions, *decide it before it is too late*.

2.1. What? Freeware, Free Software, Open-Source Software, Shareware - Unraveling the Skein

A very important issue is to distinguish clearly among what is freeware, free software, open-source software and shareware. Although there is a common misconception portrayed in many web sites and media about these terms being synonymous, they actually refer to qualitatively different legal scenarios. The importance of this question for end-users and companies becomes clear as soon as you want to distribute your digital creations: being unaware about which kind of legal situation the software you use is might potentially lead to legal liability for using such software without the required permissions (licenses). To make things tougher, there is not an unanimous opinion about the right meaning of those terms and their legal implications, so users should always read the corresponding license agreements as they are the only reliable source when it comes to legal rights and obligations. As such, the description of terms below is mostly based on commonly accepted practices within relevant software communities rather than well-established "official" definitions themselves.

By *freeware* we refer to computer software available for use at no cost or for an optional fee. Typically, freeware is fully functional and offered for an unlimited time, although some restrictions might apply. Of course, this concept can also include proprietary software provided that it is offered for free. In this sense, freeware is used to refer to software which is simply free-of-charge, with no other implications behind. Therefore, it must not be confused with *free software*, the later meaning that it can be used, studied, and modified without restriction. Although proprietary software companies typically use the term "free software" to refer to price, free software is actually a matter of freedom, not price. In words of Richard Stallman in the famous "The Free Software Definition" document [24] released by the Free Software Foundation (FSF), an organization that advocates for free software [23], to understand the concept, one should *"think of free as in free speech, not as in free beer"*.

By *open-source software* we mean computer software that is available in source code form. Usually, such source code and certain other rights normally reserved for copyright holders are provided under a software license that allows users to study, change, and improve the software. According to this concept, freeware may or may not be open-source, depending on whether or not the source code is also provided. Similarly, free software may or may not be open-source software, depending on the rights provided regarding the re-use of such software and subsequent distribution. This is however a matter of discussion. For the Free Software Foundation, free software is computer software liberally licensed to grant the right of users to use, study, change, and improve its design through the availability of its source code. From this standpoint, all licenses qualified as free software are also considered open-source licenses, but this criterion is not unanimously acknowledged.

Open-source licenses often meet (but not necessarily) the requirements of the Open Source Definition [51], used by the Open Source Initiative (OSI) [50] to determine whether a software license can be considered open-source. Such definition does not match exactly that of free software issued by the FSF. However, differences between both terms are very small, so in practice they basically refer to the same software licenses, with a few minor exceptions. According to FSF [22]: *"However, the differences in extension of the category are small: nearly all free software is open source, and nearly all open source software is free."*

Another related term is *shareware*. By it we refer to proprietary software that is provided to users for free on a trial basis only. Usually, shareware is freely provided for a limited period of time in order to offer potential customers the opportunity to use the program thus determining its usefulness and potential advantages over competitors before taking a decision about buying a license. Often shareware is also labeled as "free trial" or "trial version" to stress that meaning. In other cases, the software is offered with some limitations on functionality, such as import/export or save options and the like. Such missing functionalities can be fully activated after purchasing a license. In videogames, shareware has been traditionally used as a mean to distribute games developed by small-sized companies that do not have access to major distribution channels for their products. In general, shareware games are different than game demos in the sense that the former are much less limited in terms of playtime and number of levels. It is not uncommon that shareware games include the full game, while additional content, extras and other functionalities are only provided with the commercial license.

2.2. Software licenses

As pointed out in previous section, software can be classified according to the rights granted to end-users: availability of software at no cost, access to the source code, possibility of modifying it and distributing it and so on. All those rights are specified in the corresponding software licenses, which can be categorized in a nutshell as proprietary licenses and non-proprietary licenses. In proprietary licenses, the software publisher grants a license to use one or several copies of the software but maintains the ownership of such software so as all rights are retained by the software publisher unless otherwise specified. As a consequence, the user must necessarily accept all terms of the license in order to use the software. Typically, those terms include an extensive list of activities that users are not allowed to perform with the software, such as reverse engineering, any modification of the software, its distribution to third parties and many others.

On the contrary, in non-proprietary licenses the ownership of the copy of the software does not longer remain with the software publisher, but the end-user (different than the ownership of the copyright, that still belongs to the software publisher). As a consequence, end-user can actually use the software without accepting the license. Such acceptance is optional but it is required if end-user also wants to access to other rights such as the modification or distribution rights. At its turn, non-proprietary licenses can be essentially of two different types: copylefted or permissive. The main difference between them is that copylefted licenses state that when modified versions of such software are distributed, they must be distributed under the same terms as the original software. In particular, all improvements or modifications to copylefted software must also be distributed as free software. In other words, modified versions of software with copyleft come also with copyleft. This is sometimes referred to as "share and share alike" or "quid pro quo". The ultimate goal of copyleft is to preserve the freedom and openness of the software itself. A typical example of copyleft is the GNU General Public License [26] (GPL onwards). Under it, end-users can redistribute, reverse engineer, or otherwise modify the software, but all any modifications made and redistributed must include the source code, and the end-user is not allowed to modify the copylefted license for such new software. Additionally, if GPL code is used but not shared or sold, the code is not required to be made available and any changes may remain private. This permits developers and organizations to use and modify GPL code for private purposes without being required to make their changes available to the public.

In opposition, permissive licenses aim to give users total freedom on that software, so users can do basically anything they want with the source code, including the right to use it as a part of software released under a proprietary license. For instance, GPL requires any derivative work that is distributed to be released according to the GPL while permissive licenses, such as Berkeley Software Distribution (BSD), MIT License or University of Illinois/NCSA Open Source License do not; they only require to acknowledge the original authors. As such, permissive licenses are more free than the copylefted ones. In fact, code licensed under a permissive free software license (BSD for instance) can be incorporated into copylefted projects (for example, GPL). The new code emanating from this process becomes GPL compatible. However, the opposite is not true: GPL licensed code cannot be distributed under the BSD license without the previous consent from copyright holders. To summarize, copyleft and permissive licences are compatible, but their combination can only be distributed under the terms of the copyleft license, not the permissive licence.

A halfway between copyleft and permissive licenses is given by the GNU Lesser General Public license (LGPL) [27]. Under LGPL, copyleft restrictions apply to the program itself but they do not to other software that merely links with the program. This license is mostly used for software libraries, since LGPL libraries can be used by a non-LGPL licensed program (in fact, even by a non-GPL licensed program). A famous example of LPGL application is *OpenOffice*.

A very interesting situation is that of multiple licenses, where software is distributed under two or more different sets of terms and conditions so that end-users can choose which terms they want to use in order to further distribute the software. A typical example are some Mozilla products (such as *Firefox* web browser and *Thunderbird* e-mail client), which are actually tri-licensed, since in addition to the LGPL license, they are also GPL and MPL licensed. That MPL (Mozilla Public License) is a weak copyleft version (source code copied or changed under the MPL must stay under the MPL, but code under the MPL may be combined with proprietary files in one program) approved as a open-source license and a free software license by OSI and FSF respectively. Other famous examples are *Perl* (dual license with GPL and Artistic license) and *Ruby* (GPL dual license).

3. Open-Source and Freeware Tools for the Graphics Pipeline

In this section we provide a comprehensive (although not exhaustive) collection of open-source and freeware tools and middleware available to handle different computer graphics tasks, emphasizing their potential advantages and drawbacks with respect to their proprietary counterparts. We also provide our readers with a repository of websites and links where this freely-available software can be smoothly downloaded and installed. For the sake of simplicity, such tools are classified into the following groups:

- modeling and animation tools,
- 2D artwork,
- graphical renderers,
- audio tools,
- scripting languages,
- version-control system tools for project management and
- 3D engines.

3.1. Modeling and Animation Tools

In this group we consider software tools oriented towards the generations of models (virtual environments, objects, characters) for the virtual scenes and their animation. Among them, we select the following:

- **Blender** [6]: it is a 3D graphics open-source application released under the GPL license and arguably one of the best examples of what free software can bring to computer graphics. *Blender* is being extensively used as an open-source alternative to expensive proprietary modeling software such as *3ds Max* or *Maya*. Originally developed by Ton Roosendaal since the times of NeoGeo animation studio and Not a Number Technologies company, it is currently being developed by the Blender Foundation (chaired by Ton Roosendaal). What *Blender* offers is a suite of tools enabling the creation of interactive 3D content, with full functionality for modeling, rendering, animation, post-production and game creation and playback. The program is incredible small (with a download file size of less than 2.5MB) and with the benefits of minimal requirements in terms of hardware (a minimum of 128 MB RAM and 20 MB of free hard disk space) and cross-platform operability (with support for Windows 2000, XP and Vista, Mac OS X 10.2+, Linux 2.2.5 i386 & 2.3.2 PPC, FreeBSD 6.2 i386, Irix 6.5 mips3 and Solaris 2.8 sparc). The last stable version is *Blender* 2.49, with remarkable features for:

  - modeling (polygon meshes, NURBS surfaces, metaballs, vector fonts, Catmull-Clark subdivision surfaces, multiresolution, mesh modeling based on vertex, edge and/or face selection, organic modeling and so on),
  - keyframed animation tools including inverse kinematics, skeleton support and skinning, organic bodies, shape keys (morphing), non-linear animation, constraints, vertex weighting, soft body dynamics including mesh collision detection, Lattice-Boltzmann-methods fluid dynamics, Bullet rigid body dynamics, particle-based hair, and a particle system with collision detection,
  - nice texturing, rendering and shading effects (including cube, cylinder, sphere and view projections for texturing, support for multiple UV layers, oversampling, motion blur, UV mapping, ray tracing, fog effects, defocusing, ambient occlusion, radiosity solver, export scripts for renderers such as *Renderman*, *POVray*, *Virtuallight*, *Lux*, *Indigo* and *V-Ray*, diffuse and specular shaders, materials support, blurry reflections and refractions, normal, displacement and bump maps),
  - *Python* scripting for tool creation and prototyping, game logic, extensive support for 2D (TGA, JPG, PNG, OpenEXR, DPX, Cineon, Radiance HDR, Iris, SGI Movie, IFF, AVI, Quicktime GIF, TIFF, PSD, MOV) and 3D (*3D Studio*, AC3D, COLLADA, FBX Export, DXF, *Wavefront* OBJ, DEC Object File Format, *DirectX*, *Lightwave*, MD2, Motion Capture, Nendo, *OpenFlight*, PLY, *Pro Engineer*, Radiosity, Raw Triangle, *Softimage*, STL, TrueSpace, VideoScape, VRML, VRML97, X3D Extensible 3D, xfig) importing and exporting from other formats, task automation and custom tools,

- the subproject *Game Blender* offers powerful features for stand-alone real-time application for videogame creation, such as collision detection and dynamics simulation now supported by *Bullet* Physics Library [7] (an open-source (zlib licensed) multi-threaded 3D collision detection, soft body and rigid body physics engine for games and visual effects in film), discrete collision detection for rigid body simulations, support for vehicle dynamics (including spring reactions, stiffness, damping, tyre friction, etc.), support of all *OpenGL* lighting modes, programmable logic, audio (using the SDL toolkit) and multilayering of scenes.

All these appealing features, comparable to those of its commercial counterparts, have helped to build a solid reputation for *Blender* among media professionals and individual users. As such, it is the most advisable option for low-budget users and freelancers in what it comes to all-around modeling and animation tools. *Blender* has also shown its capabilities for ambitious projects such as the world's first and widely recognized open short movie *Elephants Dream*, followed up by open movie *Big Buck Bunny* in 2008, while a third movie is in progress.

Main drawback is probably its interface, which is limited (no drag and drop, poor intuitive tools) and confusing. In fact, *Blender* is reputed for being difficult to learn even for users familiar with other 3D graphics software and its learning path to be productive is longer than commercial packages. Documentation is also poorer; although this issue is improving lately, there is still a long way to walk to match its competing alternatives.

- **DAZ Studio** [15]: it is a modeling and animation application featuring both a rich 3D figure design and a powerful 3D animation tool. It is released by DAZ 3D Inc. [16] in two different versions: *DAZ Studio* (standard) as a freeware version and *DAZ Studio Advanced* as a shareware 30-days trial version. The last stable version is 3.0.1 and it is available for Windows (32 and 64 bits, XP or Vista recommended) and Mac OS X v.10.4+. *DAZ Studio* is a software intended for manipulation of "ready to use" posing human and non-human figures for illustrations and animation. As such, it is a convenient tool to design digital art and animation using virtual people, animals, props, vehicles, accessories, environments and more. *DAZ Studio* was created as an alternative to proprietary 3D rendering and animation shareware *Poser* [56], a tool that become very popular for digital artists creating original images featuring human figures. As opposed to *Poser*, *DAZ Studio* has been designed to provide the end-user with just the required features for the creation of imagery, while other features are included in the form of (usually commercially available) "plug-ins", which the user may add as required, thus keeping the free-of-charge core of the program into manageable size. *DAZ Studio* has been designed to be compatible with the *Poser* file formats, so it can import *Poser* models, with the exception of dynamic clothing and dynamic hair. This feature is especially valuable as it offers access to a large collection of *Poser* figures available in the market. Some of such figures are provided for free, while other are sold but they are usually inexpensive. The program has an intuitive user interface, in which you simply select your subject and/or setting, arrange accessories, setup lighting, and begin creating beautiful artwork.

- **Bryce** [8]: it is a 3D modeling, rendering and animation program originally created to generate computer images of mountains and coastlines by using fractal geometry. The program is very well suited for landscapes and advanced terrain editing as well as atmospheres and skies. Currently in version 6 as a proprietary software from DAZ 3D Inc., there is a freeware version (v5.5) available [9] (requires registration) for Windows (98, Me, 2000, NT and XP).

- **MakeHuman** [44]: it is a copyleft licensed (under GPL 3.0 terms) open-source software application to generate 3D humanoids. It is written in C++, requires *Aqsis* (see details in Section 3.3.) for rendering purposes and is available for Windows, Mac OS X and Linux, its latest stable version being 1.0 alpha5. *MakeHuman* is specifically targeted for the accurate modeling of the human form. To this aim, it includes a number of remarkable features, such as a system to simulate muscular movement and limb rotation, many facial expressions, about 3000 morphings and the possibility of mixing up different characters, a skin rendering with *Renderman* compliant engines, a new GUI (Graphical User Interface) with theme support and intuitive tabs, hair preview in 3D, export support to *Blender* and in .obj and Collada data formats (among others) and a high quality mesh optimized to work in subdivision surface model. *MakeHuman* incorporates several plugins (written in *Python*) to export a modelled and posed figure in 3D graphics formats supported by a very wide range of external modellers and rendering engines, such as Pixar's *Renderman* [64]. Thus, although *Aqsis* is the officially supported *Renderman* format renderer, export to other formats and other renderers is also provided.

- **Avimator** [4]: it is an easy-to-use, open-source (GPL licensed) editor for creating and editing avatar animations for 3D metaverse *Second Life* [66]. It is a free alternative to *Poser* and *Maya*, running on Windows, Mac OS X, and Linux platforms and built on *FLTK* (Fast, Light Toolkit) [20], a cross-platform free (LGPL licensed) GUI library, written in C++ and designed for 3D graphics programming with an interface to *OpenGL*, but still suitable for general GUI programming). *Avimator* is available for Windows, Mac OS X and Linux and complies with BVH (Biovision Hierarchy) format, a widely used character animation file format. However, the program is not longer being developed and users are adviced to try *QAvimator* instead.

- **QAvimator** [59]: it is the *Qt* port of *Avimator*, currently in alpha version, available for Windows, Mac OS X and Linux. *Qt* [62] is an application development framework widely used for the development of GUI programs as well as console tools and servers. It is written in C++ and is available for a variety of platforms, including Windows, Mac OS X, Linux and Embedded Linux, Symbian and others. The last stable version 4.6.2 is distributed under a LGPL license but depending on the version, some other license types (such as commercial, FreeQt License, Q Public license (QPL) and GPL) are also available.

- **Wings 3D** [71]: it is an open-source subdivision surface-based modeling tool available for most platforms, including Windows, Linux and Mac OS X (10.3+) under the permissive BSD license. It can be used to model and texture low to mid-range polygon models, including support for ngon meshes. In *Wings 3D* it is possible to assign materials, vertex color, UV coordinates and textures, but does not support animations and has only basic *OpenGL* rendering facilities, although it can export to external rendering software such as *POV-Ray* and *YafRay*. Because of this, it is mostly used in combination with other software more specialized in rendering and animation such as *Blender*.

- **trueSpace** [70]: it is a free all-around modeling/animation/rendering package for 3D computer graphics and animation developed by Caligari Corporation originally for Amiga in 1994 and later for Windows platform, but now owned by Microsoft. Last stable version is 7.61 released on May 2009 and it has been officially discontinued, but still some "unofficial support" is alive. Consequently, users were urged to download all free software related to this product as soon as possible.

- **Cal3D** [10]: it is a 3D skeletal character library written in C++ in a platform-/graphic API-independent way and released under the LGPL license for Windows, SGI Irix, Linux and Mac OS X platforms. Originally designed to be used in a 3D client for Worldforge (a project aimed at producing an open-source (GPL) framework for massively multiplayer online role-playing games [72]), it evolved into a stand-alone product which can be used in many different kinds of projects. Latest stable version is 0.11.0. Its architecture is comprised of two major components: the C++ library and the exporter. The C++ library provides methods to load the exported files, build characters, run animations, and access the data necessary to render them with 3D graphics, while the exporters are actually plug-ins for 3D modeling packages so that 3D artists can use the modeling tools they are more comfortable with. *Cal3D* has exporters for *Blender*, *3D Studio MAX* and *Milkshape 3D*.

- **MarbleCLAY** [45]: it is a free Japanese polygon modeler previously known as *Etude3D*. Currently in version beta 5.8a, it can be downloaded for Windows (registration required). A MarbleSDK toolkit (version beta 5.6) for developers is also available.

- **QuARK (Quake Army Knife)** [61]: it is a free and open-source (GPL licensed) program for developing 3D assets for a large variety of video games, mostly first-person shooters using engines similar to or based on the *Quake* engine (a game engine designed to power blockbuster *Quake* game [60]; it uses BSP (binary Space partitioning) and is released under the GPL license), although other game engines (such as *Source*, *Genesis3D*, *Crystal Space* or *Torque*) are also supported. Its nice integration of a map editor, model editor, archive editors and texture management allows users to directly edit maps and can import, export, manipulate and convert models, sounds, textures and various other game assets, or create any of these assets from scratch by using a brush-based editor. It offers a textured view where maps can be rendered in three different modes: wireframe, solid color and textured. It is quite popular, with more than 30 games (including famous best-selling games such as *Call of Duty, Doom, Half-Life, medal of Honor, Quake, Soldier of Fortune, Star Trek, Star Wars* or *Team Fortress*) and a countless number of modifications (mods) supported. Last version available so far is 6.6.0 beta 3.

- **Deled** [17]: it is a free all-in-one 3D modeler and level-editor for Windows oriented towards game development and specifically designed to create static objects/worlds. Developed by Delgine [18], it provides tools for geometry editing, animation, UV mapping, light mapping and ray tracing along with great support for commonly used file formats (.obj, .d3d, .dbo, .raw, Collada, .3ds, etc.) and game engines.

3.2. 2D Artwork

- **GIMP (GNU Image Manipulation Program)** [25]: it is a multilingual cross-platform (available for Windows, Mac OS X (under X11, with a native version in experimental stage), Linux, Solaris, FreeBSD) free software (GPL licensed) raster graphics editor. Originally created for UNIX systems and later migrated to other major OS, last stable version 2.6.8 is written in C and GTK+ (the object-oriented *GIMP* toolkit). Although it is primarily used for photo retouching, image composition and image authoring, *GIMP* is an all-around graphics program in what concerns image manipulation and editing. As such, it can be used as a simple paint program (with several ways of selecting colors, different kinds of custom brushes and patterns, nice capacities for image editing and modification), an expert quality photo retouching program (with a large provision of layers, layer masks and channels), an online batch processing system, a mass production image renderer, an image format converter (supporting a number of different file formats, including .bmp, .gif, .jpeg, .mng, .pcx, .pdf, .png, .ps, .psd, .svg, .tiff, .tga, .xpm, and many others) and so on. It is also extensible, supporting advanced scripting capabilities (*Scheme*, *Python*, *Perl*) and with over 100 plug-ins already available. It also supports animation in a frame-as-layer format. Although *GIMP* was initially considered only for simple tasks and amateur users, it is now capturing the attention of professionals looking for a free alternative to commercial software, notably *Adobe Photoshop*. Although recent reports state that *GIMP* is not yet powerful enough to be a sufficient replacement for high-end commercial tools, significant steps are being done and *GIMP* is slightly gaining acceptance in the professional market.

- **Krita** [40]: it is a cross-platform free (GPL licensed) raster graphics editor included with the KDE-based *KOffice* suite. KDE [38] is a free software community that produces a set of multi-platform programs and applications, including the *Qt*-based KDE desktop environment that became specially popular in Linux (now in version 4.0 and called *Plasma* [55]). KDE community releases *KOffice* [39] as a free open-source (GPL, LGPL and BSD licenses) office suite available for Windows, Linux and Mac OS X. *KOffice* contains a number of suite components such as a word processor (*KWord*), a spreadsheet application (*KSpread*), a presentation program (*KPresenter*) and several other programs including *Karbon14* [37] (a GPL-licensed vector graphics editor to create clipart, logos, illustrations or photorealistic vector images), and *Krita* (a bitmap graphics editor, primarily designed as a painting program, with some image processing features). *Krita* is very well-suited for sketching and painting, and emphasizes the creation of digital painting images from scratch (such as concept art, creation of comics and textures for rendering) as opposed to manipulating existing photographs. Current stable version of the program is 2.1.0.

- **Inkscape** [29]: it is a multilingual open-source (GPL licensed) cross-platform (available for Windows, Mac OS X - under X11, although the GTK+ toolkit can be compiled to run natively under Quartz - and UNIX) vector graphics editor application. Although it is focused on being fully compliant with the XML, SVG, and CSS open standards, the process is still incomplete. *Inkspace* originated as a forked project of open-source (PGL licensed) Sodipodi project [67], whose primary native format was open standard SVG and is now discontinued. Written in C++ (using GTK+), *Inkscape* is especially popular on Linux environments. Currently *Inkscape* can officially import SVG, SVGZ, AI, and PDF and export SVG, SVGZ, PDF, PostScript, EPS, EPSi, LaTeX and *POVRay*. Some formats have additional support through Inkscape extensions, including PDF, EPS, *Adobe Illustrator*, Dia and Sketch. Notably, text rendering is based on the open-source (LGPL licensed) *Pango* library [52], used by software developers and corporations (including Mozilla) to render text in high quality, emphasising support for multilingual text. This allows *Inkscape* to support several complex scripts in languages such as Arabic, Thai or Tibetan.

- **xNormal** [73]: it is a free open-source graphical application to generate normal, ambient occlusion, displacement and relief maps. It also includes an interactive 3D viewer with multiple mesh and textures format support, shaders and realtime soft shadows and glow effect, and is provided with a complete and easy-to-use C++ SDK to write plugins and extend the program. *xNormal* is used by amateurs, artists and in projects, mostly videogames (*Fragfist, Darkest of Days, Wing Commander Vega Strike*).

3.3. Graphical Renderers

- **Aqsis** [1]: it is a cross-platform free rendering suite (under the GPL, with some parts under the LGPL) currently in version 1.6.0, compliant with the *Renderman* standard. It focuses on stability and production usage and includes features such as constructive solid geometry, depth-of-field, extensible shading engine (DSOs), instancing, level-of-detail, motion blur, NURBS, procedural plugins, programmable shading, subdivision surfaces, subpixel displacements and more.

- **Pixie** [54]: it is an open-source (under GPL and LGPL licences) *Renderman*-compliant ray-tracing renderer for generating photorealistic images. It compiles for Windows (using Visual Studio 2005), Linux and on Mac OS X (using Xcode or Unix-style configure script). It is based on the Reyes rendering architecture, but also support ray-tracing for hidden surface determination. Its last stable version is 2.2.6.

- **POV-Ray (Persistence of Vision Raytracer)** [57]: it is a free photo-realistic rendering program based on the popular ray-tracing technique and developed for various computer platforms (in fact, any platform with a compatible C++ compiler). This program has been very popular in academic and image production amateur environments, because of the simplicity of the program, the high-quality of the output images, its conceptual approach to modeled objects (all primitive objects are described in *POV-Ray* by mathematical functions instead of polygonal meshes, so they are truly mathematical objects, and hence accurate), the large collection of resources and support from third parties (including tutorials, models, scenes, textures, examples and the like) and the availability of the source code, that happened well before it became a common practice. For this reason, the program is distributed with a *POV-Ray* license that allows free distribution of the program source code and binaries, but restricts commercial distribution and the creation of derivative works other than fully functional versions of *POV-Ray* (in this sense, it is not an open-source software according to OSI). Current stable version is 3.6.

- **RayShade** [63]: it is a free and extensible system for creating ray-traced images. It is written in C, yacc, and lex, and runs on many different platforms. Originally developed at Princeton University at late 80s, *Rayshade* is very easy to use: it simply reads a description of a scene to be rendered and produces a color image corresponding to the description. The last stable version is 4.0.6.

- **YafaRay** [74]: it is a free, open-source (released under the LGPL license) ray-tracing program integrated into the 3D modelling software *Blender*. It means that it can be used to render scenes made within *Blender* directly, without the need for an exporter. *YafaRay* is based on predecessor program *YafRay*, but it is a completely rewritten software fully developed using C++ and that uses an XML scene description language. *YafaRay* has a modular structure, with a kernel connected with the other components: scene loader, lights and shaders. This modularity along with an API, allows development of rendering plug-ins, for using *YafaRay* from other programs such as *Wings 3D*. Its architecture gives it a great portability and there are versions for Windows, Mac OS X and Linux. The last stable version is 0.1.1.

- **LuxRender** [43]: it is a free, open-source (GPL licensed) cross-platform (Windows, Mac OS X, Linux) software rendering system for image synthesis. *LuxRender* simulates the flow of light according to physical equations, thus producing realistic images of photographic quality. In addition, it fully supports high-dynamic range (HDR) rendering. The program is merely a 3D rendered, meaning that all content to be rendered must be generated by using an external program. Fortunately, the program has fully functional exporters for *Blender* and *Maya*, while exporters for *Cinema4D*, *XSI* and *3D Studio* are in progress. Depending on the kind of scene to be rendered, different rendering algorithms are applied, such as bidirectional path tracing combined with Metropolis sampling for indoors and other scenes or complex lighting and path tracing for simple scenes and outdoors. By using light groups, users can output various light situations from a single rendering, or make adjustments to the balance between light sources in real time. For each light source, intensity and colour can be adjusted on the fly. *LuxRender* features a variety of material types, such as matte, glossy and physically accurate representations of metals and glass. Complex properties such as absorption, dispersive refraction and thin film coating are also available. Last stable version is 0.6.1.

- **DrQueue** [19]: it is a free, open-source (GPL licensed) software tool primarily used to manage a render farm. It is used for a range of applications across the visual effects industry (mostly for animations used as visual effects in films and advertising) and for general batch processing jobs in science and engineering. *DrQueue* provides distributed render queueing on a per-frame basis and management of these tasks and is available for several platforms, including Windows, Mac OS X, Linux, FreeBSD and Irix. The application comprises three main tools: master, slave and drqman. The master acts as a central server, where all tasks are stored, while the slave software is run on each node in the cluster and it reports its status back to the master periodically. Typically, a task is composed of jobs distributed to those slave nodes via a script. Finally, drqman is a GUI used for job control and monitoring. *DrQueue* supports several applications, such as *3Delight, 3DSMax, After Effects, Aqsis, Blender, BMRT, Cinema 4D, Lightwave, Luxrender, Mantra, Maya, Mental Ray, Nuke, Pixie, Shake, Terragen, Turtle, V-Ray* and *XSI*. Last stable version is 0.64.3.

3.4. Audio Tools

- **Audacity** [3]: it is a very popular and top-downloaded free, open-source (GPL licensed) cross-platform (available for Windows, Mac OS X, Linux and BSD) multilingual (with more than 20 languages supported) digital audio editor and recording application. It supports importing and exporting WAV, AIFF, MP3 (via LAME), Ogg Vorbis and all file formats supported by LGPL-licensed *libsndfile* library, as well as other formats such as WMA, AAC, AMR and AC3, via the optional LGPL-licensed *FFmpeg* library. Last stable version is 1.2.6.

- **Ardour** [2]: it is a free (GPL licensed) hard-disk recorder and digital audio workstation application. It is written in C++ and is available for Linux, Mac OS X and FreeBSD. Its goal is to provide digital audio workstation software suitable for professional use and its recording capabilities are limited only by the hardware where is is installed. It supports an arbitrary number of tracks and busses, dragging, trimming, splitting and timestretching recorded regions with sample-level resolution and can be used as an audio mastering environment. Import and export functionalities are available for more than 30 audio file formats. Its last stable version is 2.8.7.

- **MPlayer** [46]: it is a cross-platform (Windows, Mac OS X, Linux, Unix-like systems) free, open-source (GPL licensed) media player. It supports a wide variety of media formats, including audio (AAC, AC3, ALAC, AMR, DTS, FLAC, Intel Music Coder, Monkey's Audio, MP3, Musepack, RealAudio, Shorten, Speex, Vorbis, WMA, Bink), video (Cinepak, DV, H.263, H.264/MPEG-4 AVC, HuffYUV, Indeo, MJPEG, MPEG-1, MPEG-2, MPEG-4 Part 2, RealVideo, Sorenson, Theora, WMV, Bink), subtitles (AQTitle, ASS/SSA, CC, JACOsub, MicroDVD, MPsub, OGM, PJS, RT, Sami, SRT, SubViewer, VOBsub, VPlayer) and image (BMP, JPEG, MNG, PCX, PTX, TGA, TIFF, SGI, Sun Raster) formats. It can also be used to display TV from a TV card, play and capture radio channels or save all streamed content to a file. *MPlayer* is a command line application that supports different optional GUI frontends for each of its supported operating systems. Last stable version is 1.0rc3.

- **FluidSynth** [21]: it is a free open-source (GPL, LGPL licensed) program which synthesizes using SoundFont technology without need for a SoundFont-compatible soundcard. The size of loaded SoundFont banks is limited by the amount of RAM available. It can be used for live audio synthesis of MIDI events or for rendering MIDI files to disk, using SoundFont instruments. It can also be embedded in other applications. The software is available for Linux and Windows. The Linux version has a GUI written in C++ around the Qt4 toolkit called *qsynth* (beta version) that is also open-source (GPL-licensed).

3.5. Scripting Languages

- **Perl** [53]: it is a cross-platform, free (GPL licensed, Artistic license also available) high-level, interpreted, dynamic programming language. It was created by Larry Wall in 1987 as a general-purpose scripting language for UNIX originally developed for text manipulation, with some features influenced by C, AWK and sed. Now, *Perl* is used for a wide range of tasks including system administration, web development, network programming, games, and GUI development. It is a very pragmatic language, with emphasis on efficiency and easiness to use rather than in elegance, and it supports multiple programming paradigms (procedural, object-oriented, and functional styles are supported). *Perl* is part of the three P's (*Python* and *PHP* being the other two) as the most popular dynamic languages for Web applications. It is also extensively used to communicate systems and interfaces not specifically designed to operate with each other. Last stable version of the language is 5.12.0.

- **Python** [58]: it is a cross-platform, free (Python Software Foundation license), general-purpose, high-level dynamic programming language created by Guido van Rossum at the end of the 80s. *Python* supports multiple programming paradigms, primarily object-oriented, but also imperative and (to a lesser extent) functional programming and aspect-oriented programming. *Python* is a very extensible language; it actually comes with a small core of functionalities that can readily be extended with new modules written in C, C++ or *Cython* (a programming language created to simplify writing C modules for *Python*). *Python* is often used as a scripting language for web applications as well as for 3D animation packages (such as *Maya, MotionBuilder, Softimage, Cinema 4D, BodyPaint 3D* and *Blender*), 2D imaging programs (*GIMP, Inkscape, Paint Shop Pro*) and several videogames. It is also commonly used in many other non-scripting tasks, for instance, as an extension language for existing modules and applications that need a programmable interface. The last stable version of *Python* is 3.1.2.

- **Lua** [42]: it is a free (MIT licensed), cross-platform, multi-paradigm (scripting, imperative, functional and object-oriented) programming language. *Lua* was designed and developed by members of the Computer Graphics Technology Group at the Pontifical Catholic University of Rio de Janeiro (Brazil) to be simple, small, portable, fast, and easily embedded into applications. It is also an "extensible extension language"; the extension language refers to the fact that *"it helps to extend applications through conguration, macros, and other end-user customizations. Lua is designed to be embedded into a host application so that users can control how the application behaves by writing Lua programs that access application services and manipulate* *application data."* [28]. *Lua* is extensible because is provided as a small core that can be extended with user functions written in both *Lua* and C. Because of these appealing features and its small learning curve, *Lua* is now widely used as a scripting language in the computer graphics and videogame industries. In fact, it has arguably become the most popular scripting language for game development, with many remarkable titles using it, such as *Baldurs Gate, Escape from Monkey Island, FarCry, Grim Fandango, Homeworld 2, Illarion, Impossible Creatures, Psychonauts, The Sims* and *World of Warcraft*. Last stable version of *Lua* is 5.1.4.

- **Ruby** [65]: it is a free (GPL and Ruby licensed), cross-platform (Windows, Mac OS X, Linux, UNIX, Symbian) dynamic, general-purpose object-oriented programming language that combines syntax inspired by *Perl* with *Smalltalk*-like features. It was originally developed in 1995 by Yukihiro Matsumoto with the aim to create *"a scripting language that was more powerful than Perl, and more object-oriented than Python"*. Indeed, *Ruby* supports multiple programming paradigms, including functional, object oriented, imperative and reflective. It is also designed to minimize user's effort by doing the most intuitive and expected action. *Ruby* syntax is quite similar to those of *Perl* and *Python*, while its semantics is clearly object-oriented, since every data type is an object and every function is a method. Last stable version of *Ruby* is 1.9.1.

3.6. Version-Control System Tools for Project Management

A version-control system (VCS) software is responsible for the management of changes to documents, programs, and other information stored as computer files. It is most commonly used in software development, where a team of people may change the same files. As such, they are essential tools for the organization of multi-developer projects. In this section, we describe some of the most popular open-source VCS.

- **CVS** [14]: it is a free, open-source (GPL licensed) version-control system tool for open-source code. *CVS* become very popular in the open-source community in the 90s, although it was replaced in users' preferences by *Subversion* and recently by other tools such as *Bazaar*, *Git* or *Mercurial*. *CVS* is written in C and available for Windows and Unix-like platforms. It uses a client-server architecture, where typically these two components are connected by a LAN or Internet. Last stable version is 1.11.23.

- **Apache Subversion** [69]: formerly known as just *Subversion*, it is a free, open-source (Apache licensed) version-control system tool initiated in 2000 as a continuation and strong improvement of *CVS*. As the project advanced significantly, it was accepted for Apache incubator and recently as a top-level Apache project. *Subversion* is highly recognized by its reliability, the simplicity of its model and usage and its ability to cover the needs of a wide variety of users and projects, ranging from individuals to large-sized companies and corporations. Consequently, it has been widely accepted not only in the free software and open-source communities, but also in corporative world for many multi-developer projects. Its latest stable version is 1.6.11.

- **Bazaar** [5]: it is a free, open-source (GPL licensed), cross-platform (with versions for Windows, Mac OS X and major GNU/Linux distributions) distributed (no central server required) VCS. Written in *Python*, its commands are quite similar to those of *CVS* and *Subversion*. In fact, one of major *Bazaar*'s goals is to be user-friendly and task-efficient. *Bazaar* is not a purely distributed VCS; instead, it supports working with or without a central server. Changing from an existing central version control tool to *Bazaar* does not require to change their workflow. Furthermore, it is possible to use both methods at the same time with the same project. In addition, *Bazaar* is well compatible with other VCS: team members can continue to commit exactly as they currently do with *CVS* or *Subversion*, making it possible to migrate to a distributed revision control using *Bazaar* without radically changing the former project structure until the team becomes ready to go fully distributed. *Bazaar* also allows for interoperation with many other systems (including *CVS, Darcs, Git, Perforce, Mercurial*) by allowing to import/export the history. The program has a plug-in architecture (with more than 100 plug-ins already developed) making it easily extensible. Users can develop new functionalities via a *Python* API, making it easy to embed in tools and to integrate with existing infrastructure. Integration via XML is also possible. Last stable version is 2.1.1.

3.7. 3D Engines

- **OGRE (Object-Oriented Graphics Rendering Engine)** [47]: it is a free (MIT licensed, with LGPL license with some exclusions for versions 1.6 or earlier), cross-platform (with full support of *OpenGL* [48] and *Direct3D* graphics libraries and versions for Windows, Mac OS X and Linux distros), scene-oriented, flexible 3D rendering engine designed to make it easier and more intuitive for developers to produce applications by taking advantage of the powerful features of last-generation hardware-accelerated 3D graphics. Written in C++, *OGRE* is designed to provide a general world-class graphics solution that can be effectively used for games, simulations, business applications and others, rather than being a specialized tool for specific tasks. To this aim, it comes with a basic cores of routines, while specific needs (such as sound, networking, Artificial Intelligence, collision, physics) can be solved by linking *OGRE* with other libraries or programs. Though it also comes with other facilities (vector and matrix classes, memory handling, etc.), they are considered supplemental; the emphasis is on being a rendering engine. *OGRE* has an object oriented design with a plugin architecture that allows easy addition of features, thus making it highly modular. The rationale is that *OGRE* does not assume what type of game, application or demo you want to make. Accordingly, it uses a flexible class hierarchy allowing you to design plugins for specialized tasks so as to allow you to make any kind of scene at will. There exist a number of *OGRE* bindings to other languages and frameworks including *Perl*, *PureBasic*, Python-OGRE for *Python*, Ogre.rb for *Ruby*, Ogre4j for Java and OgreDotNet, GMOGRE for *Game Maker* and MOGRE for .NET. Another remarkable feature of *OGRE* is the extensive set of consistent documentation (including tutorials, manuals, books, reference guides, a lovely wiki, case studies, external resources) that allows the users to get the most with less. Its very active community of developers and users does not certainly hurt either. Last stable version of *OGRE* is 1.7.1 (codename Cthugha).

- **Irrlicht** [33]: it is a free, open-source (zlib licensed, a permissive free software license which defines the terms under which the zlib [75] and libpng [41] software libraries can be distributed. It has been approved by FSF as a free software licence and by OSI as an open-source license), cross-platform (with support for Windows, Mac OS X, Linux and Windows CE and portable to other systems including the Xbox, PlayStation Portable, SymbianOS and iPhone) high-performance real-time 3D engine written and usable in C++. Originally started in 2003 by Nikolaus Gebhardt, *Irrlicht* features a powerful high level API for creating complete 3D and 2D applications such as games or scientific visualizations, providing high-performance real-time 3D rendering using *OpenGL* and *Direct3D*. The engine comes with a library of standard material renderers, allowing fallback materials where user hardware is unable to handle advanced techniques although new materials can be added to the engine at run-time, allowing users to meet their needs by writing their own. The engine also provides support for collisions, a mix of indoor/outdoor scenes, a terrain renderer, sky domes and boxes, bones for meshes, shadows, particle systems, billboards, water surfaces, a nice GUI with support for mouse, keyboard and joystick, a XML reader and writer called *irrXML* [36], and several extensions such as *irrEdit* World Editor [30], contains a powerful radiosity lightmap generator and a scripting interface using *Squirrel* [68] scripts (a high level imperative, object-oriented programming language, designed to be a light-weight scripting language that meets the size, memory bandwidth, and real-time requirements of applications like video games and distributed as an open-source (zlib licensed) software), *irrKlang*, the Irrlicht audio library created to overcome the limitation that original Irrlicht engine does not support sound by itself, and two extensions by Chris Mash: *IrrPhysx* [35] (and Nvidia PhysX wrapper library specifically designed for *Irrlicht*, currently in progress with a beta version available) and *IrrAI* [31] (an open-source generic AI module accounting for various Artificial Intelligence behaviors commonly found in video games, also in progress). The engine supports a myriad of formats, including JPEG, PNG, TGA, BMP, PCX, PPM, PSD and WAL for texture files, and .b3d, .x, .ms3d, .md3, md2, .irr, .irrmesh,3ds, .lwo, .xml, .dae, .mesh, .my3d, .lmts, .bsp, .dmf, .oct, .csm, .stl, and .ply for animated and static mesh files. There are also several language bindings (see [34] for details) which make the engine available to other languages such as *C#*, *VisualBasic*, *Delphi*, *Java*, *.NET*, *Perl*, *Ruby*, *Python*, *FreeBASIC*, *Lua*, *C++ Builder* and *Game Maker*. *Irrlicht* is reputed by its small size and compatibility with several hardware. It also has a large supporting community and a comprehensive, well-organized documentation both online and in printed form. Last stable version of *Irrlicht* is 1.7.1.

- **OpenSceneGraph** [49]: it is a multi-platform (Microsoft Windows, Mac OS X, Linux, IRIX, Solaris and FreeBSD), open-source (LGPL-based OpenSceneGraph Public License), high-performance 3D graphics toolkit, used by application developers in fields such as visual simulation, computer games, virtual reality, scientific visualization and modelling. The toolkit is written in standard C++ using *OpenGL*, and provides support for performance increasing features such as view frustum, small feature and occlusion culling, LOLs (levels of detail), *OpenGL* fast paths and latest extensions, multi-threading and configurable support for multiple CPU/multiple GPU machines, database optimization, particle effects, a wide range of 2D and 3D formats, framebuffer objects, pbuffers and frame buffer render-to-texture effects. Last stable version is 2.8.2.

- **Crystal Space** [13]: it is a free (LGPL licensed), cross-platform (Windows, GNU/Linux, Mac OS X), full-featured software development kit (SDK) providing real-time 3D graphics for applications such as games and virtual reality. It is typically used as a game engine but the framework is more general and can be used for any kind of 3D visualization. It encompasses two main components: *Crystal Space* (a modular, configurable, and extensible rendering engine supporting *OpenGL* and advanced features such as shaders and lighting systems, physics, 3D sounds, animation blending, foliage, terrain, virtual file system, physical peripherals, and more) and *CEL* [11] (an entity system supporting higher-level functionality, such as the runtime package environment *CELstart* [12], generic event system, avatar and camera management, artificial intelligence (behavior trees, path finding, neural networks and genetic algorithms), vehicles, and more). One popular way to make *CELstart* applications is with *Blender* through the *blender2crystal* script. It is possible to make full *CELstart* games from within *Blender*. *Crystal Space* is programmed in C++ and is very modular, with several independent plug-ins available. The client programs use the plug-ins, like the *OpenGL 3D* renderer, by registering them via *Crystal Space*'s Shared Class Facility (SCF). Last stable version of *Crystal Space* is 1.4.0.

4. Conclusion

This chapter explores the on-going process of "democratization" in the field of computer graphics as a consequence of the recent appearance of powerful freeware and open-source tools for almost all tasks of the graphics pipeline. The chapter discusses some issues related to this new approach, such as the kind of licenses available and their implications for further use. We also provide pointers to a large collection of open-source and freeware tools and middleware available to handle just about every development tasks. Such tools are described and classified in order to provide our readers with a repository of websites and links of freely-available software. Some hints to help our readers to use the appropriate software for specific tasks are also reported.

It is authors' opinion that this "democratization" process, although yet vigorous and widely accepted, is still in its primary steps. Many freeware and open-source tools are (at different extent) not as powerful as their commercial counterparts, or lack important technical or documentation features. These limitations have discouraged several end-users to adopt open alternatives, in spite of their evident benefits. As open-source and free software is gaining increasing reputation, more human effort and resources are being allocated in order to improve such features. This process runs in parallel with the adoption of open tools in other computer science disciplines, so we foresee a back-and-forth flow of mutual enrichment between open-source computer graphics tools and open-source computer science tools. It is our belief that this process is still in its infancy and promising, exciting new projects and tools will arise everywhere. Although commercial software will still play an important role for large-sized projects, we envision a further popularization of freeware and open-source tools amongst small and medium-sized projects and individual users for years to come. *It will be an exciting process for sure!*

Acknowledgments

The authors would like to thank Prof. Frank Columbus for his kind invitation to write this chapter and to all staff of Nova Publishers for their diligent work towards the publication of this contribution.

This research has been supported by the Computer Science National Program of the Spanish Ministry of Education and Science, Project Ref. #TIN2006-13615 and the University of Cantabria.

References

[1] Aqsis web site: *http://www.aqsis.org/*

[2] Ardour web site: *http://www.ardour.org/*

[3] Audacity web site: *http://audacity.sourceforge.net/*

[4] Avimator web site: *http://www.avimator.com/*

[5] Bazaar web site: *http://bazaar.canonical.com/en/*

[6] Blender web site: *http://www.blender.org/*

[7] Bullet web site: *http://www.bulletphysics.org/*

[8] Bryce web site: *http://www.daz3d.com/i.x/software/bryce/*

[9] Bryce v5.5 (freeware): *http://www.daz3d.com/i/support/downloads?product=bryce*

[10] Cal3D web site: *http://home.gna.org/cal3d/*

[11] Crystal Space's CEL web site: *http://www.crystalspace3d.org/main/CEL*

[12] Crystal Space CELStart web site: *http://www.crystalspace3d.org/main/CELstart*

[13] Crystal Space web site: *http://www.crystalspace3d.org/*

[14] CVS web site: *http://www.nongnu.org/cvs*

[15] DAZ Studio web site: *http://www.daz3d.com/i/3d-models/-/daz-studio-3?item=8969&_m=d*

[16] DAZ 3D Inc. web site: *http://www.daz3d.com*

[17] Deled web site: *http://www.delgine.com/index.php?filename=product_deled*

[18] Delgine web site: *http://www.delgine.com*

[19] DrQueue web site: *http://www.drqueue.org/cwebsite/*

[20] FLTK web site: *http://www.fltk.org/*

[21] FluidSynth web site: *http://fluidsynth.sourceforge.net/*

[22] The Free Software Foundation: *http://www.gnu.org/philosophy/categories.html*

[23] The Free Software Foundation Web site: *http://www.fsf.org/*

[24] The Free Software Definition: *http://www.gnu.org/philosophy/free-sw.html*

[25] GIMP web site: *http://www.gimp.org/*

[26] The GNU General Public License v3.0: *http://www.gnu.org/licenses/gpl-3.0.txt*

[27] The GNU Lesser General Public License: *http://www.gnu.org/copyleft/ lesser.html*

[28] Ierusalimschy, R., Figueiredo, L. H., Celes, W: *The evolution of Lua*. Proc. of ACM SIGPLAN conference on History of programming languages. San Diego, USA,. pp. 2.1-2.26 (2007).

[29] Inkscape web site: *http://www.inkscape.org/*

[30] IrrEdit web site: *http://www.ambiera.com/irredit/*

[31] IrrAI web site: *http://sites.google.com/site/chrisjmash/irrai*

[32] IrrKlang web site: *http://www.ambiera.com/irrklang/*

[33] Irrlicht web site: *http://irrlicht.sourceforge.net/*

[34] Irrlicht bindings web site: *http://irrlicht.sourceforge.net/links.html*

[35] IrrPhysx web site: *http://sites.google.com/site/chrisjmash/irrphysx*

[36] IrrXML web site: *http://www.ambiera.com/irrxml/*

[37] Karbon14 web site: *http://www.koffice.org/karbon/*

[38] KDE project web site: *http://www.kde.org/*

[39] KOffice web site: *http://www.koffice.org/*

[40] Krita web site: *http://krita.org/*

[41] libpng library web site: *http://libpng.org/*

[42] Lua web site: *http://www.lua.org/*

[43] LuxRender web site: *http://www.luxrender.net/*

[44] MakeHuman web site: *http://www.makehuman.org/*

[45] MarbleCLAY web site: *http://homepage3.nifty.com/escargot/MCLFrm.html*

[46] MPlayer web site: *http://www.mplayerhq.hu/*

[47] OGRE web site: *http://www.ogre3d.org/*

[48] OpenGL web site: *http://www.opengl.org/*

[49] OpenSceneGraph web site: *http://www.openscenegraph.org/*

[50] The Open Source Initiative Web site: *http://opensource.org/*

[51] The Open Source Definition: *http://opensource.org/docs/osd*

[52] Pango web site: *http://www.pango.org/*

[53] Perl web site: *http://www.perl.org/*

[54] Pixie web site: *http://www.renderpixie.com/*

[55] Plasma web site: *http://www.kde.org/workspaces/plasmadesktop/*

[56] Poser web site: *http://poser.smithmicro.com/poser.html*

[57] POV-Ray web site: *http://www.povray.org/*

[58] Python web site: *http://www.python.org/*

[59] QAvimator web site: *http://www.qavimator.org/*

[60] Quake game web site: *http://www.idsoftware.com/games/quake/quake/*

[61] QuARK web site: *http://quark.sourceforge.net/*

[62] Qt web site: *http://qt.nokia.com/*

[63] Rayshade web site: *http://www-graphics.stanford.edu/ cek/rayshade/rayshade.html*

[64] Renderman web site: *https://renderman.pixar.com/*

[65] Ruby web site: *http://www.ruby-lang.org/*

[66] Second Life web site: *http://secondlife.com/*

[67] Sodipodi project web site: *http://sodipodi.sourceforge.net/*

[68] Squirrel web site: *http://squirrel-lang.org/*

[69] Subversion web site: *http://subversion.apache.org/*

[70] trueSpace web site: *http://www.caligari.com/*

[71] Wings 3D web site: *http://www.wings3d.com/*

[72] Worldforge project web site: *http://www.worldforge.org/*

[73] XNormal web site: *http://www.xnormal.net/*

[74] YafaRay web site: *http://www.yafaray.org/*

[75] zlib library web site: *http://zlib.net/*

In: Computer Graphics
Editor: Martin J. Davis

ISBN: 978-1-61761-811-6

Chapter 6

DATA REPRESENTATION FOR SCIENTIFIC VISUALIZATION: AN INTRODUCTION

***Dan R. Lipşa*[1]* *Robert S. Laramee*[2]† *R. Daniel Bergeron*[3]‡ *and Ted M. Sparr*[4]§**
[1]Swansea University, Wales, UK
[2]Swansea University, Wales, UK
[3]University of New Hampshire, Durham, NH, USA
[4]University of New Hampshire, Durham, NH, USA

ACMS COMPUTING CLASSIFICATION SYSTEM I.3.6 [Computer Graphics]: Methodology and Techniques; H.2.8 [Database Management]: Database applications–Scientific databases

Keywords: sampling and reconstruction of data, Discrete Fourier Transform, frequency domain, Nyquist rate, low pass filters, convolution operation, wavelets transforms

1. Introduction

Most would agree that we live in an age characterized by an explosion in data and information. The very rapid increase in computing power often described using Moore's law has enabled scientists, researchers and practitioners to collect, store and analyze unprecedented amounts of data. Tools that enable insights into these large quantities of data are of ever increasing importance.

Visualization is an important field of study that enables users to explore, analyze and present large amounts of data rapidly. Visualization as a branch of computer science is expanding and evolving quickly in response to the current data explosion. This is evident in the rapid increases in both commercial and open source visualization tools [14] as well

*E-mail address: csdan@swansea.ac.uk
†E-mail address: E-mail address: r.s.laramee@swansea.ac.uk
‡E-mail address: rdb@cs.unh.edu
§E-mail address: tms@cs.unh.edu

as literature [11, 4]. Even Google has introduced a visualization API [3]. What we present is an introduction to the field of scientific visualization from a data-centric point of view. This paper provides the following contributions and benefits:

- We provide a concise introduction and a logical starting point for those interested or new to scientific visualization.
- We provide a description of scientific data, its characteristics and ways to model the data e.g. various grid representations
- Various filtering and interpolation methods that operate on and enhance the data are described.
- A brief introduction to both the theory and practice of data sampling and reconstruction is provided.
- Wavelets and wavelets transforms, an important mathematical tool for building multiresolution representations of data are introduced.

The resulting manuscript provides the reader with a concise and valuable introduction to scientific visualization starting with a data centric point of view. We aim to provide an educational tool for those new to the topic. The rest of this manuscript is organized as follows: the next section presents a brief description of scientific data characteristics and common processing. Those motivate the next sections: we present common types of scientific datasets and some of their storage methods, we briefly describe the theory behind the sampling and reconstruction of data points from a continuous function and we present the main concepts of wavelets and wavelets transforms.

2. Characteristics and common processing of scientific data

A scientific dataset consists of spatial data values either collected from the real world or produced by a computer simulation. Several different attributes (for instance the concentration of several chemical elements) can be acquired or produced for each point in space and these measurements can be repeated over a period of time. Scientific datasets have different characteristics based on the spatial arrangement of their data points: they differ in how they are stored and in what algorithms can be used to process them. We present common types of scientific datasets and some of their storage methods.

Scientists explore scientific datasets in order to discover features of interest or to construct and study models of real world phenomena. Query operations are used to restrict the explored region of data, and visualization algorithms are used to display the data. A value for an attribute at a point in space can be thought of as being a sample from a function with values in every point in $\mathbb{R}^3$ where $\mathbb{R}$ is the set of real numbers. Often we need attribute values at other points in space than the sample data points contained in the dataset. The theory behind the sampling and reconstruction of data points from a function is summarized.

Often scientific datasets are very large, much larger than the main memory of a computer. Because of large disk-drive latency, visualization algorithms designed to process data from main memory cannot be directly applied to data stored on disk. One way to deal with large scientific datasets is to use a lower resolution version of the dataset for query, visualization and exploration. This can be done by using multiresolution (MR) and adaptive resolution (AR) representations of the dataset.

A multiresolution (MR) representation of the dataset consists of a hierarchy of versions of the original dataset, each having a different resolution. Typically a user starts by exploring the coarsest resolution version, which is much smaller than the original dataset. Higher resolution versions of the dataset are used either when the user zooms in locally to view a region of interest or when the user stops the exploration thus providing more time to render a higher resolution version of the dataset.

An adaptive resolution (AR) representation partitions a dataset into regions of different resolutions. Ideally, the resolution for each region is determined such that the error for that region is smaller than a user specified *error tolerance* for the dataset. A region of similar values will have a low resolution while a region with larger variations will have a high resolution such that the error for both regions will be smaller than the error tolerance specified for the dataset. The error for a region at the original resolution is zero. The error for a region at a lower resolution than the original is calculated by comparing the region at the original resolution with the region at the lower resolution.

Wavelets are a popular mathematical tool used for building a multiresolution representation of scientific data, image compression and in many other areas of computer graphics. We present the main concepts of wavelets and wavelets transforms.

3. Scientific Data Representation and Storage

In this section we present a model for scientific data. Based on the relationship between neighboring data points, scientific datasets can be represented as structured or unstructured grids. These are also described in this section.

3.1. A Data Model

Rhodes et al. [5] present a formal data model for scientific data which we briefly summarize in the next few paragraphs.

Scientific datasets represent a phenomenon defined over a continuous domain D. These datasets store values for a measured or simulated quantity that describes the phenomenon. Measurements are done and samples are recorded only for a finite number of points from the continuous domain D. If $\Delta \subset D$ is the set of sample points, the set of values stored in the dataset is given by a function $f_\Delta : \Delta \to \Omega$ where Ω is a subset of V, and V is the set of all possible values that the measured quantity can have. The error in each sample point is defined as a function $E_\Delta : \Delta \to E$ where E is the set of possible error values. Errors can appear because of the measurement devices or because of approximations and errors in the simulation. Formally, the dataset is represented [5] as a tuple:

$$R = \langle \Delta, \Omega, f_\Delta, E_\Delta \rangle \tag{1}$$

where Δ the set of all sample points, Ω the set of possible values for the measured quantity, f_Δ the function that gives the values measured at any sample point and E_Δ the function that gives the error at any sample point. The positions of all sample points is called the *geometry* of the dataset.

Data points in scientific datasets are normally part of a grid which is a tiling (tessellation) of the n-dimensional space, and the data model presented so far does not make provisions for that. Finding the neighbors of a data point and using tiles (cells) for processing the dataset is commonly used in scientific visualization so Rhodes et al. augment their model to contain a grid. The new model L which adds a grid component τ called the *topology* of the dataset to the previous model is presented in Equation (2).

$$L = \langle R, \tau \rangle \tag{2}$$

The scientific dataset model presented so far, which contains both the position in space of every sample point (the geometry of the dataset) and the grid information (the topology of the dataset) does not provide a description of the phenomenon measured over the whole continuous domain D over which the phenomenon occurs. To extend the measurements in the sample points to the whole domain D the authors use two *interpolation* functions. They use f_D to calculate the measured value in other points besides the sample points and they use E_D to calculate the error in other points besides the sample points. To calculate the value at any point in the domain D the interpolation function uses values in the sample points which are neighbors of that point. Both geometric and topological information may be used to do that. The new model is presented in Equation (3).

$$M = \langle L, f_D, E_D \rangle \tag{3}$$

When describing a grid of data points, there are two characteristics that are important: the structure of the grid which specifies the neighborhood information (topology) and the mapping between the structure and the position in space of each point (geometry). There are two main types of grids: structured grid and unstructured (irregular) grid. In the interest of clarity, we present all the concepts in this section for two-dimensional data but they apply equally well to three-dimensional data.

3.2. Structured Grids

A structured grid of data points can be represented as a two-dimensional array, each position in the array storing all attribute values for a point. The coordinates in space of a data point can be calculated from its position in the array, together with some additional information that depends on the grid type. The neighbors of a data point can be retrieved implicitly from the position of the point in the array. These two characteristics lead to significant space saving when storing a structured grid dataset in memory or in a file.

Because it maps directly to a two-dimensional array, structured grid data is normally stored in a file using *linear storage*, by traversing its indexes (axes) in predefined order using nested loops [6]. To optimize disk access, a two-dimensional array is often stored in a file using *chunked storage* when data is split in tiles (chunks, cubes or bricks) of equal size, and each individual tile is stored contiguously in the file using linear storage. Tiles are stored in the file in linear fashion by traversing the axes of the volume in a certain order using nested loops. The order of traversing the axes and the size of the tiles is determined by the expected access pattern of the application.

Table 1. a. Regular grid ($d_x \neq d_y$), b. cartesian grid ($d_x = d_y$), c. rectilinear grid ($d_x^i \neq d_x^{i+1}, d_y^i \neq d_y^{i+1}$).

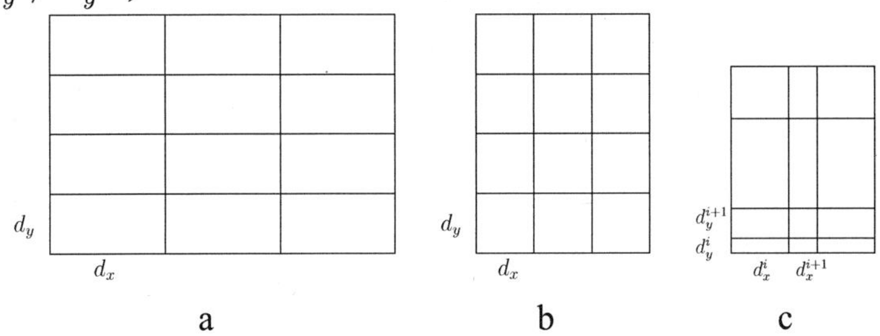

With the same neighborhood information (structure) there can be different grid types based on the position in space of the data points. To specify the position in space of every point in the dataset we need to specify the position in space of the point at the origin of the array besides other information that depends on the type of structured grid that is used for the dataset. There are four different types of structured grids: regular, cartesian, rectilinear and curvilinear.

On a *regular grid* all data points are located on a tiling (tessellation) of the space with a rectangular tile. To specify the position in space of all points in the dataset, the additional information we need is the size (d_x, d_y) of the tile. Figure 1-a shows a two-dimensional regular grid.

A *cartesian grid* is a special case of a regular grid where all sides of the tile have the same length (i.e. $d_x = d_y$). To specify the position in space of all points in the dataset, the additional information we need is the length of a side of the square tile. Figure 1-b shows a two-dimensional cartesian grid.

Rectilinear grids have all data points on a tiling of the space with rectangular tiles of different size. These rectangles are specified by intersections of lines perpendicular on X and Y axes. All lines perpendicular to the X-axis are specified with an array of tile side lengths along X-axis and the same is true for all lines perpendicular to the Y-axis. So, to specify the position in space of all the points of the dataset, the additional information needed is two arrays of lengths, one for each axis X and Y. Figure 1-c shows a two-dimensional rectilinear grid.

To understand a *curvilinear grid* we can think of a rectilinear grid with flexible edges, where the vertices of the grid are not in the original positions but are moved in space. It is possible for a curvilinear grid to have shared boundaries, for instance a 2D rectilinear grid that is wrapped around a cylinder. Sometimes, curvilinear grids specify the position in space of its points using a function of the point position in the structure array. It is also common for the position information to be stored explicitly in each point. Figure 1 shows a curvilinear grid (on the left) and a cartesian grid that has the same topological structure as the curvilinear grid (on the right).

3.3. Unstructured or Irregular Grids

An unstructured (irregular) grid data starts with data points at arbitrary positions in the two-dimensional space. To visualize data it is essential to have neighborhood (structure)

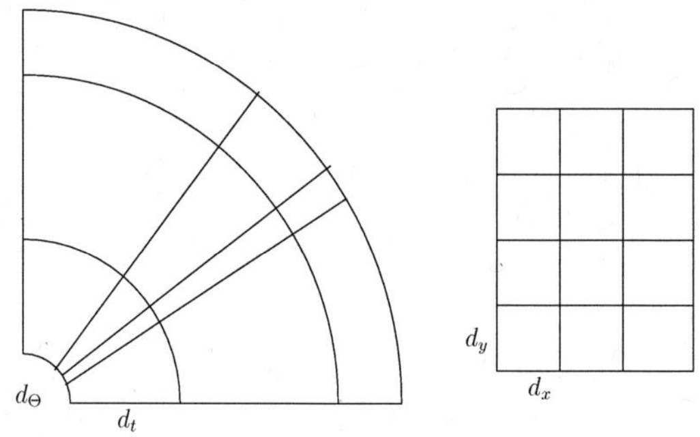

Figure 1. A curvilinear grid and a cartesian grid with the same topological structure ($d_t \rightarrow d_x, d_\Theta \rightarrow d_y$).

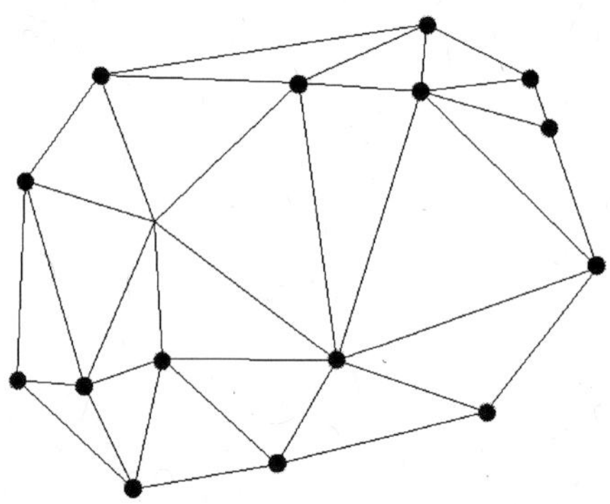

Figure 2. An unstructured (irregular) grid dataset

information for the data points which is usually created with a procedure called triangulation. A triangulation of a set of points in the plane is obtained by adding the maximum set of edges that connect two points such that no new edge can be added without intersecting existing edges.

The data points together with the imposed structure determines a tiling of the two-dimensional space where each tile is a triangle. Both the position of points in space and neighborhood information needs to be stored together with data to enable efficient processing of irregular data.

Irregular volume data is usually stored in a format called *index cell set* (ICS) [7] as a list of vertices and a list of tetrahedral cells. For each vertex we store the x, y, z coordinates in space of that vertex and all data attributes. Each cell contains four indexes (references) to vertices in the vertex list.

4. Sampling and Reconstruction of Data

Often, visualization algorithms are used to process data obtained by sampling a function defined in all points in space. Ideally, the sampled function value, should allow us to reconstruct the original function without any loss, but often this is not possible. We would like to know how many samples we need from the original function such that reconstruction without loss is possible and how to reconstruct the signal such that we minimize the loss. The answers to these questions are provided by the field of signal processing [2]. In the rest of this section we present properties of functions of one variable (which can represent time or space) but the results we present can be extended to three or four dimensional functions that are used in scientific visualization.

4.1. Discrete Fourier Transform (DFT) and the Inverse DFT

An important tool in studying sampling and reconstruction of functions is Fourier analysis [1, 8, 12] which allows a function to be expressed as a (possibly infinite) sum of sinusoids of different frequency, amplitude and phase. In practice, the frequency, amplitude and phase for those sinusoids is calculated using the Discrete Fourier Transform (DFT). Suppose we sample a function $x(t)$ at $t_0, t_1, ..., t_{N-1}$ to get N sample values $x_0, x_1, ..., x_{N-1}$. From the sample values we can define N sinusoids using the DFT formula:

$$X_k = \sum_{n=0}^{N-1} x_n e^{-i\omega_k t_n} \tag{4}$$

In Equation (4) $k = 0, \ldots, N-1$, x_n is the sample value for $t_n = nT$ the nth sampling instant, T is the sampling interval, X_k is the amplitude and phase for $\omega_k = \frac{2\pi k}{N} f_s$ the kth frequency sample and $f_s = 1/T$ is the sampling frequency. If x is a function in the temporal domain, its Fourier transform X is said to be the representation of the function x in the frequency domain. The Fourier transform of a signal is a complex function of the form $X_k = R_k + iI_k$ that encodes both the amplitude $|X_k| = \sqrt{R_k^2 + I_k^2}$ and the phase $\phi_k = \tan^{-1} \frac{I_k}{R_k}$ of the sinusoid with frequency ω_k.

The DFT formula is obtained by viewing the N signal samples as an n-dimensional vector in the vector space $\mathbb{C}^N$, where $\mathbb{C}$ is the set of complex numbers. In this space the set of vectors $s_1, s_2, \ldots, s_N$ is an orthogonal base where $s_k(n) = e^{i\omega_k t_n}$ is the complex sinusoid with frequency ω_k. The amplitude and phase X_k in the DFT formula is obtained by projecting vector x onto the kth complex sinusoid s_k. All original signal samples x_n can be obtained by adding together all projections onto vectors s_k that form a base of $\mathbb{C}^n$. This transformation is called the inverse DFT:

$$x_n = \frac{1}{N} \sum_{k=0}^{N-1} X_k e^{i\omega_k t_n} \tag{5}$$

The complex sinusoid s_k can be understood by using the Euler identity $e^{i\omega_k t_n} = \cos \omega_k t_n + i \sin \omega_k t_n$. Complex sinusoid s_k contains two sinusoids, one for the real and one for the imaginary axes of the complex plane. Note that both $\sin$ and $\cos$ can be thought of as sinusoids because $\cos \theta = \sin(\theta + \pi/2)$.

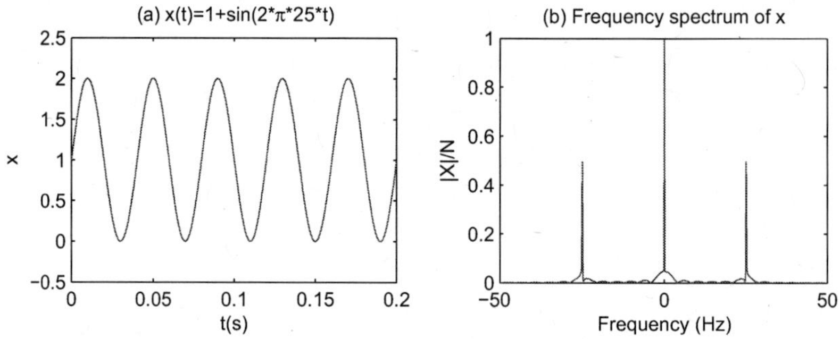

Figure 3. Frequency spectrum of a sin function: (a) $x(t) = 1 + \sin 2\pi 25t$ and (b) frequency spectrum of x, where $X = \mathrm{DFT}(x)$ and N is the number of samples.

4.2. Graphical Representation of Functions in the Frequency Domain

Radian frequencies [8] $\omega_k = \frac{2\pi k}{N} f_s$ with $k = 0, 1, \ldots, N-1$ create N equally spaced frequency samples in the interval $[0, 2\pi f_s)$ with values:

$$0, 2\pi\frac{1}{N}f_s, 2\pi\frac{2}{N}f_s, \ldots, 2\pi\frac{N/2-1}{N}f_s, 2\pi\frac{N/2}{N}f_s, \ldots, 2\pi\frac{N-1}{N}f_s \qquad (6)$$

You can add or subtract a multiple of $2\pi f_s$ from these radian frequencies without changing their meaning because $e^{i(\omega_k + 2\pi f_s)t_n} = e^{i\omega_k t_n} e^{2\pi f_s t_n}$. But $e^{2\pi f_s t_n} = e^{2\pi \frac{1}{T} T n} = e^{2\pi n} = 1$. An equivalent list of frequency samples obtained by subtracting $2\pi f_s$ from all frequencies greater or equal to $2\pi\frac{N/2}{N} f_s$ is:

$$0, 2\pi\frac{1}{N}f_s, \ldots, 2\pi\frac{N/2-1}{N}f_s, \underbrace{2\pi\frac{-N/2}{N}f_s, \ldots, 2\pi\frac{-1}{N}f_s}_{\text{negative frequencies}} \qquad (7)$$

The list of frequencies in Equation (7) can be reordered as:

$$\underbrace{-\pi fs, -\pi(1-\frac{2}{N})fs, \ldots, -\pi\frac{2}{N}fs}_{\text{negative frequencies}}, 0, \pi\frac{2}{N}, \ldots, \pi(1-\frac{2}{N})fs$$

The representation of a signal in frequency domain is usually shown with frequencies in the interval $[-\pi f_s, \pi f_s)$, where a negative frequency can be translated to a frequency in the interval $[\pi f_s, 2\pi f_s)$ as shown above. When the Fourier transform of a function x is displayed graphically, the phase ϕ_k is usually ignored and the amplitude $|X_k|$ is showed as a function of frequency ω_k. Figure 3 shows the graphs for $x(t) = 1 + \sin 2\pi 25t$ and for the DFT(x). Note that the DFT graph shows a zero frequency (DC - direct current) component which is equal to 1 and two complex sinusoids with frequency equal to -25 and 25 Hz and amplitude 0.5. The two complex sinusoids combine to yield a real sinusoid with frequency of 25 Hz and amplitude of 1. Note that for real signals x we have that $|X(\omega_k)| = |X(-\omega_k)|$ for all frequencies ω_k so the graphical representation of X_k is symmetric about axis Y. The

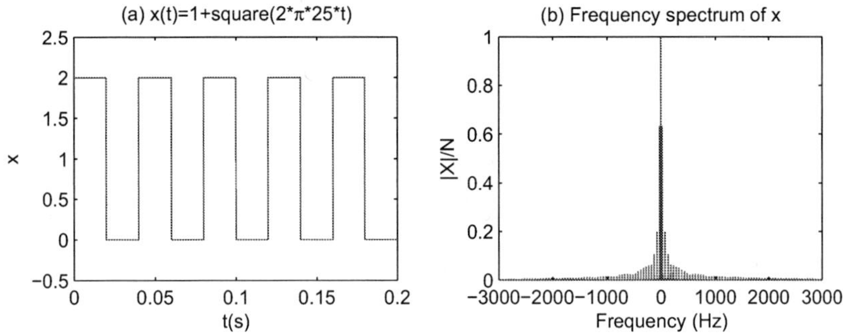

Figure 4. A square function and its frequency spectrum. (a) $x(t) = 1 + \text{square}\ (2\pi 25t)$ and (b) frequency spectrum of x, where $X = \text{DFT}(x)$ and N is the number of samples.

amplitude of the real sinusoid is twice the amplitude of $|X(\omega_k)|$. This can be explained by using the Euler identity to express a real sinusoid as a sum of two complex sinusoids with the same absolute frequency and half the its amplitude:

$$\cos\theta = (e^{i\theta} + e^{-i\theta})/2 \quad \text{and} \quad \sin\theta = (e^{i\theta} - e^{-i\theta})/(2i)$$

4.3. The Nyquist Rate

It has been shown [8] that a signal can be reconstructed completely from its samples if the signal was sampled at a frequency that is greater than $2 * f_h$, where f_h is the highest frequency component in the signal. That minimum sampling frequency is called the *Nyquist rate*. Unfortunately, many signals in the real world have infinite frequency spectrum which means that those signals cannot be reconstructed from a set of samples, regardless of the sampling frequency. For instance, a square wave has infinite frequency spectrum because its value changes discontinuously as showed in Figure 4.

4.4. Low Pass Filters and the Convolution Operation

An operation that is often useful, called low pass filter, removes all components with frequencies larger than a certain frequency ω from a signal. This operation makes it possible to sample and reconstruct the remaining signal without loss because its frequency spectrum is finite. A low pass filter in the frequency domain is realized by multiplying the signal in frequency domain with a pulse function

$$p(k) = \begin{cases} 1 & \text{if } |\omega_k| < \omega \\ 0 & \text{otherwise} \end{cases}, \text{where } k = 0..N-1$$

where N is the number of samples.

An image can be thought of as a function f of two variables where the color of the pixel at position (x, y) is given by $f(x, y)$. A low pass filter in the frequency domain on function f causes blurring in the associated image as this filter removes sharp transitions in a signal.

Figure 5 shows the signal $x(t) = 1 + \text{square}\ (2\pi 25t)$ limited at 500 Hz in the frequency domain. To be able to reconstruct the remaining signal without loss we have to sample the

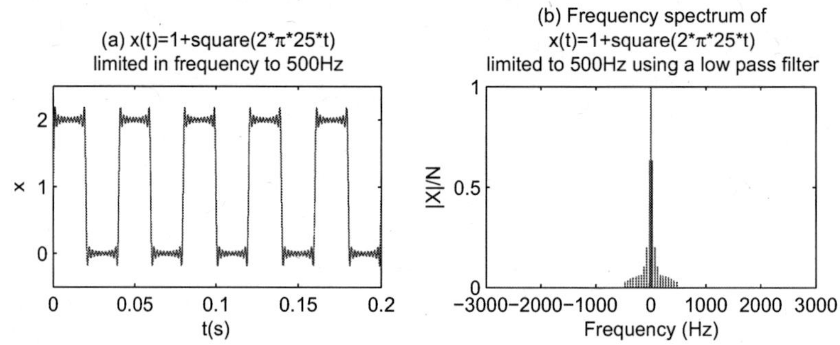

Figure 5. A square function ($x(t) = 1 + \text{square}\ (2\pi 25t)$) limited in frequency, (to 500 Hz) represented in time and frequency domains. Plot (a) show the time domain and plot (b) shows the frequency domain.

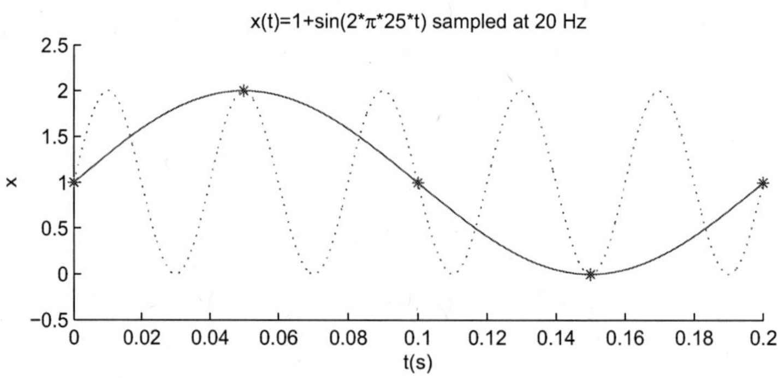

Figure 6. Aliasing: a signal sampled at frequency under Nyquist rate, can look like a lower frequency signal. In the figure $x(t) = 1 + \sin 2\pi 25t$ (interrupted line) is sampled at 20 Hz while its Nyquist rate is 50 Hz. Samples look as if they are part of a sinusoid with frequency 5 Hz ($1 + \sin 2\pi 5t$ drawn with a continuous line)

signal at a sampling rate above the Nyquist rate, which is 1000 Hz. If the sampling rate for a signal is below the Nyquist rate higher frequency components in the signal can masquerade as lower frequency components, a phenomenon called *aliasing*. Figure 6 shows a sinusoid sampled at below twice its frequency. The samples obtained look like a sinusoid with lower frequency than the original.

To apply a low pass filter to a signal x we need to multiply X, the representation of the signal in the frequency domain, with a pulse function. Signal processing theory shows that multiplication in the frequency domain of X with a function Y corresponds to $x * y$ in the time domain, where $*$ is an operation called convolution and x and y are the Inverse Fourier Transform of signals X and Y respectively. For discrete signals, the convolution between signal x of length n and signal y of length m is a signal w of length $m + n - 1$. Algebraically, the convolution is the same operation as multiplying the polynomials whose

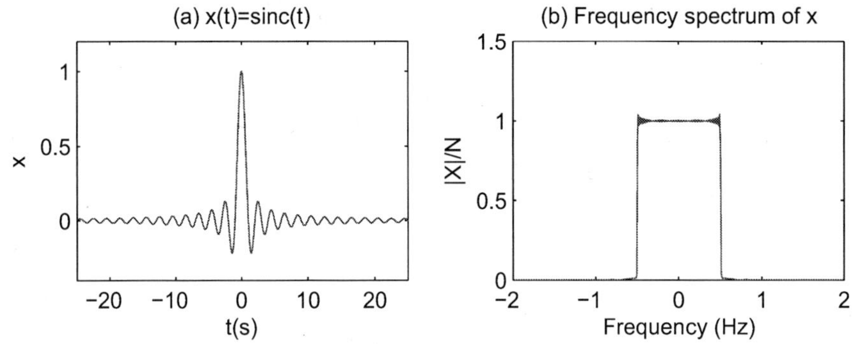

Figure 7. A low pass filter in the frequency domain, and its representation in the time domain, the sinc function. (a) $x(t) = \text{sinc}(t)$ and (b) the pulse function, sinc representation in the frequency domain. To obtain a perfect pulse function in the frequency domain, x has to be transformed using the Discrete Fourier Transform over $(-\infty, \infty)$.

coefficients are elements of x and y.

$$w(k) = \sum_j x(j)y(k-j) \quad \text{where } k = 0, \ldots, m+n-2$$

and the sum is over all the values which lead to legal subscripts for x and y.

4.5. Reconstruction Filters

It has been shown [13] that the Inverse Fourier Transform of a pulse function is a function called sinc where $\text{sinc}(t) = \frac{\sin \pi t}{\pi t}$. That means that to apply a low pass filter to a function in the frequency domain we need to convolve the function with a sinc function in the temporal domain. Figure 7 shows a sinc function together with its frequency spectrum.

Unfortunately, sinc has infinite domain, so in practice, the sinc function is approximated using a pulse, a triangle or a Gaussian function. Figure 8 shows a pulse, triangle and Gaussian functions in the temporal domain and in the frequency domain.

Suppose that a signal has its frequency spectrum limited so that a sample from the signal can be theoretically used to reconstruct the original signal without loss. This reconstruction can be done if the signal is sampled at a frequency twice as large as its largest frequency component. It can be shown that the frequency spectrum of the sample is obtained by duplicating the frequency spectrum of the original signal at equally spaced frequencies along the entire frequency spectrum. To reconstruct the original signal, the sample has to be multiplied with a low pass filter in the frequency domain or convolved with a sinc function in the temporal domain. We note that sinc has infinite domain so, in practice, the signal will be convolved with one of its approximations which has finite domain. That means that, in practice, the original signal cannot be accurately reconstructed even if sampling was done at above Nyquist rate. Differences between the original signal (frequency spectrum limited) and the reconstructed signal are called *artifacts*.

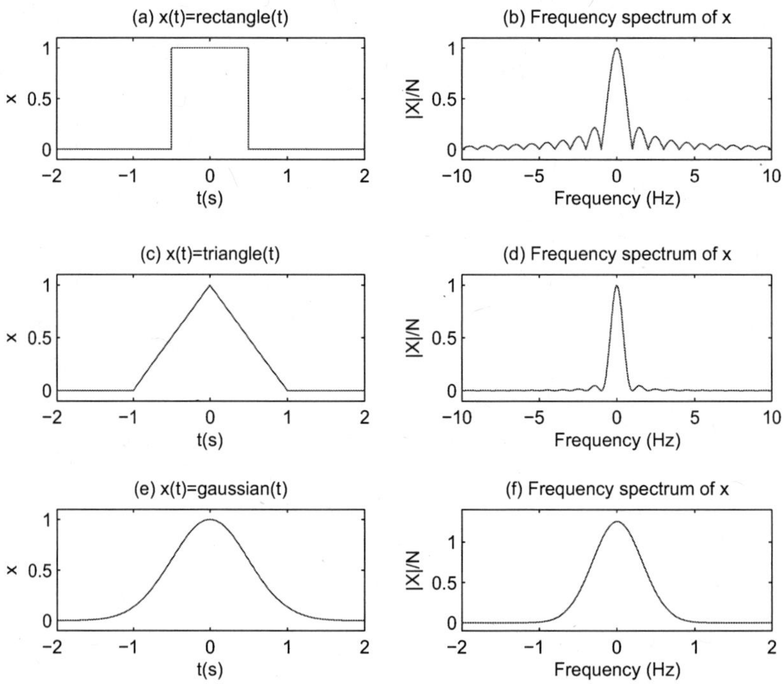

Figure 8. Approximations of the low pass filter (pulse function) in the frequency domain and their representations in the time domain: rectangle, triangle and Gaussian functions. The time domain is represented in (a), (c) and (e) and the frequency domain is represented in (b), (d) and (f).

5. Wavelets Transforms

Wavelets [9, 10] are a mathematical tool for decomposing data into approximation and detail constituents. This decomposition can be applied recursively which yields a hierarchy of approximations to the original data from the original high resolution to a desired low resolution. Each of these approximations, together with detail data can be used to completely recover the original data. There are different kinds of wavelets which determine different ways of decomposing a dataset and can be applied to different kind of data such as an image, a curve, a surface or a volume. Wavelets are used in many areas of computer graphics such as image compression, level-of-detail control for editing, rendering surfaces and global illumination [10].

The computation that transforms data into approximation and detail components is called an *analysis filter* or a *decomposition filter* and the computation that recovers the original data from approximation and detail data is called a *synthesis filter* or a *reconstruction filter*.

As an example we apply an *analysis filter* to a unidimensional dataset to decompose it into an approximation part and a detail part. We are going to use the *Haar analysis filter*, a simple and widely used filter. Suppose that we start with a dataset with four values $[5, 3, 7, 9]$. To obtain the approximation part we average every two values in the list to get

$[\frac{5+3}{2}, \frac{7+9}{2}]$ which is $[4, 8]$. To obtain the detail part we subtract every two values in the list and then we divide the result by two to get $[\frac{5-3}{2}, \frac{7-9}{2}]$ which is $[1, -1]$. From a dataset with four values we obtain an approximation dataset that has two values and a detail dataset that has two values. We can apply our filter again on the approximation dataset with two values to get an approximation value and a detail value. The entire process is summarized in Table 2:

Table 2. Haar analysis filter

Resolution	Approximation	Detail
4	$[5, 3, 7, 9]$	
2	$[4, 8]$	$[1, -1]$
1	$[6]$	$[-2]$

The one approximation value for the dataset followed by detail values in order of increasing resolution is called the *Haar wavelet transform* of the dataset. For our example the wavelet transform is $[6, -2, 1, -1]$. Note that using the wavelet transform, we can reconstruct any level of resolution including the original data.

To decompose a 2D dataset (for example an image), the Haar decomposition filter is generalized in two dimensions. The 1D filter is run on all rows of the dataset and then the 1D filter is run on all columns of the horizontal decomposition resulted in the previous step. This yields the average data stored in the upper left quadrant of the 2D dataset and detail data stored in the rest of the quadrants. The process is continued recursively, on the average data. (the next data that is split is the upper left quadrant). The Haar decomposition filter is generalized for 3D data in a similar fashion.

An alternate view of a sequence of values is to view it as a piece-wise constant function defined on the interval $[0, 1)$ with values in the set of real numbers. For example, a sequence with two values can be seen as a function which has two constant values over intervals $[0, 1/2)$ and $[1/2, 1)$. The set of all functions with two values is denoted with V^1 (2^1 is the number of values that a function in the set can take). A sequence with four values can be seen as a function which has four constant values over intervals $[0, 1/4)$, $[1/4, 1/2)$, $[1/2, 3/4)$, $[3/4, 1)$ and the set of all functions with four values is denoted with V^2 (2^2 is the number of values that a function in the set can take). A sequence with 2^j values can be seen as a function which has constant values over equal intervals of size $1/2^j$ and the set of all functions with 2^j values is denoted with V^j.

Each set V^j can be thought of as a vector space, where each function with 2^j values is a vector in this space. A basis for this vector space is the following set of scaled and translated "box" functions:

$$\phi_i^j = \phi(2^j x - i). \qquad i = 0, \ldots, 2^j - 1.$$

where the box function ϕ is defined by:

$$\phi(x) = \begin{cases} 1 & \text{for } 0 \leq x < 1 \\ 0 & \text{otherwise} \end{cases}$$

For example, the basis for V^2 is showed in Figure 9. The function used in our previous

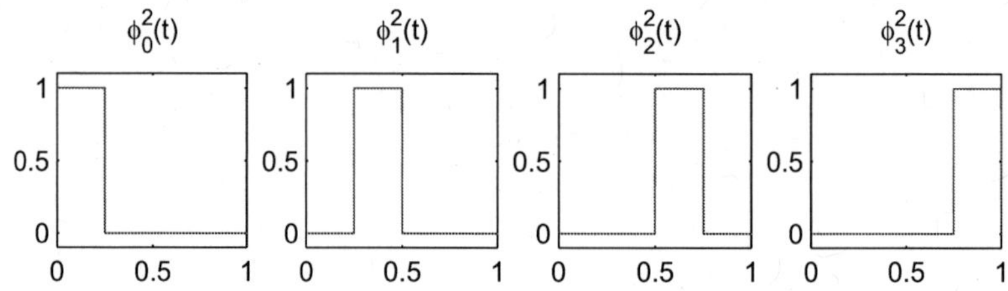

Figure 9. Any sequence of four values can be seen as a function that has four constant values over intervals $[0, 1/4), [1/4, 1/2), [1/2, 3/4)$ and $[3/4, 1)$. Each of these functions, in turn, can be seen as a vector in a vector space denoted with V^2. This figure shows a basis for V^2 formed by scaled and translated box functions

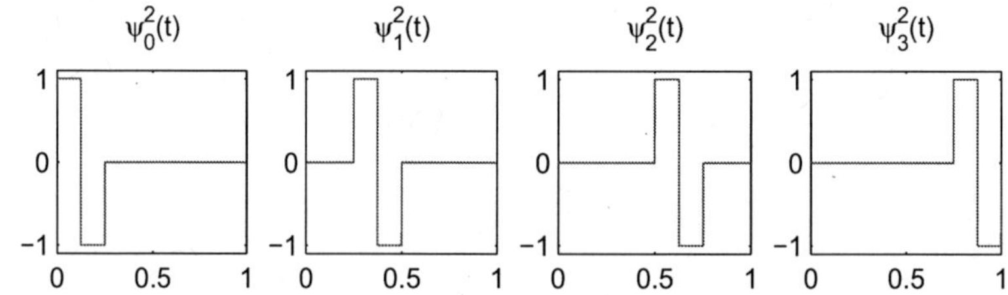

Figure 10. Haar wavelets for W^2 or basis for vector space W^2. W^2 is the complement of V^2 (vector space of functions with 4 values) in V^3 (vector space of functions with 8 values) so $V^2 \cup W^2 = V^3$

example $[5, 3, 7, 9]$, can be expressed in terms of V^2 basis as: $f = 5\phi_0^2 + 3\phi_1^2 + 7\phi_2^2 + 9\phi_3^2$.

The set V^j of all functions with 2^j values is included in the set V^{j+1} of functions with 2^{j+1} for all values j. So we have:

$$V^0 \subset V^1 \subset \ldots \subset V^j \subset V^{j+1} \qquad \text{for all } j \geq 0$$

We define the inner product between two functions f and g in the vectors space V^j as the integral of the product of the two functions: $\langle f, g\rangle = \int_0^1 f(x)g(x)\mathrm{d}x$. This can be used to define vectors in V^j that are orthogonal to each other, as the vectors for which the inner product is zero. We can now define a set, denoted with W^j, which is the orthogonal complement of V^j in V^{j+1}. This means that $V^j \cup W^j = V^{j+1}$ and every vector in W^j in orthogonal to every vector in V^j. A basis for W^j, known as the Haar wavelets are given by:

$$\psi_i^j = \psi(2^j x - i), \qquad i = 0, \ldots, 2^j - 1$$

where

$$\psi(x) = \begin{cases} 1 & \text{for } 0 \leq x < 1/2 \\ -1 & \text{for } 1/2 \leq x < 1 \\ 0 & \text{otherwise} \end{cases}$$

For example the Haar wavelets for W^2 are showed in Figure 10. The decomposition presented in Table 2 can be thought as a change of basis in vector space V^2. We start with the box functions basis: $f = 5\phi_0^2 + 3\phi_1^2 + 7\phi_2^2 + 9\phi_3^2$. We express the vector in V^2 in terms of the bases for V^1 and W^1: $f = 4\phi_0^1 + 8\phi_1^1 + 1\psi_0^1 + (-1)\psi_1^1$. Then, we express the vector in V^1 ([4, 8]) in terms of the bases for V^0 and W^0: $f = 6\phi_0^0 + (-2)\psi_0^0 + 1\psi_0^1 + (-1)\psi_1^1$. This is the Haar wavelet transform of the original function.

The Haar wavelet transform can be extended in two and three dimensions. For example in two dimensions we can apply the Haar filter on rows and then apply the Haar filter on columns to get an approximation that is one fourth of the size of the original data plus detail coefficients that are three fourths of the size of the original data. The process continues until we get a value which is an approximation of the entire dataset and detail values.

6. Conclusions

We have provided a concise introduction into the field of scientific visualization from a data-centric point of view. We have presented scientific data characteristics and common processing and those motivated the next topics of our manuscript. We have described a formal data model and common types of data representation and storage for scientific data. We have briefly presented the theory behind sampling and reconstruction of data. Wavelets and wavelets transforms, a common way to build a multiresolution hierarchy for dealing with large data was introduced. We hope to have provided a student or researcher new to the field of scientific visualization with an understanding of fundamental concepts used in the field, and a good starting point for further study.

References

[1] James D. Foley, Andries van Dam, Steven K. Feiner, and John F. Hughes. *Computer Graphics: Principles and Practice*, chapter 14, pages 617–646. Addison-Wesley, New York, NY, USA, 1996.

[2] R.C. Gonzalez and R.E. Woods. *Digital Image Processing, Third Edition*, chapter 4. Pearson Prentice Hall, Upper Saddle River, NJ, USA, 2008.

[3] Google. Google Visualization API, 2008. online document, accessed Jul. 2009, published Mar. 2008, http://code.google.com/apis/visualization.

[4] C. Hansen and Editors C. Johnson. *The Visualization Handbook*. Elsevier Academic Press, Boston, MA, USA, 2005.

[5] Philip J. Rhodes, R. Daniel Bergeron, and Ted M. Sparr. A Data Model for Distributed Multiresolution Multisource Scientific Data. In *Hierarchical and Geometrical Methods in Scientific Visualization*, Tahoe City, CA, USA, 2002. Springer-Verlag.

[6] Sunita Sarawagi and Michael Stonebraker. Efficient Organizations of Large Multidimensional Arrays. In *Proc. of the Tenth International Conference on Data Engineering*, pages 328–336, Washington, DC, USA, 1994. IEEE Computer Society.

[7] C. Silva, Y. Chiang, J. El-Sana, and P. Lindstrom. Out-of-Core Algorithms for Scientific Visualization and Computer Graphics, Course Notes for Tutorial 4. In *IEEE Visualization*, Boston, MA, USA, 2002. IEEE Computer Society Washington, DC, USA.

[8] Julius O. Smith. *Mathematics of the Discrete Fourier Transform (DFT) with Audio Applications, Second Edition*. W3K Publishing, Standford, CA, USA, 2007. online book, accessed Feb. 12 2008, http://ccrma.stanford.edu/ jos/mdft/.

[9] EJ Stollnitz, AD DeRose, and DH Salesin. Wavelets for computer graphics: a primer. *IEEE Computer Graphics and Applications*, 15(3):76–84, 1995.

[10] E.J. Stollnitz, T.D. DeRose, and D.H. Salesin. *Wavelets for Computer Graphics: Theory and Applications*. Morgan Kaufmann, San Francisco, CA, USA, 1996.

[11] A. C. Telea. *Data Visualization, Principles and Practice*. A. K. Peters, Ltd., Wellesley, Massachusetts, USA, 2008.

[12] Larry N. Thibos. *Fourier Analysis for Beginners*. Visual Sciences Group, Bloomington, IN, USA, 2003. online book, accessed Sept. 05 2008, http://research.opt.indiana.edu/Library/FourierBook/toc.html.

[13] Larry N. Thibos. *Fourier Analysis for Beginners*, chapter 11. Volume 1 of *1* [12], 2003. online book, accessed Sept. 05 2008, http://research.opt.indiana.edu/Library/FourierBook/toc.html.

[14] F.B̃. Viegas, M. Wattenberg, F. van Ham, J. Kriss, and M. McKeon. Many Eyes: A Site for Visualization at Internet Scale. *IEEE Transactions on Visualization and Computer Graphics,*, 13(6):1121–1128, 2007.

In: Computer Graphics
Editor: Martin J. Davis

ISBN: 978-1-61761-811-6

Chapter 7

A SURVEY ON THE GPU COMPUTING REVOLUTION

M. Martínez-Zarzuela, [*] ***R. Cabido-Valladolid,***
A. Sanz-Montemayor and F.J. Díaz-Pernas
University of Valladolid and University Rey Juan Carlos (Spain)

Abstract

In recent times, Graphics Processing Units (GPUs) are considered not only for graphics, but also for speeding-up the execution of general purpose algorithms that can be expressed following a stream processing model. When GPUs became programmable, the scientific community noticed that the enormous computational power behind these processors could be exploited to accelerate applications in many research fields. As a result, relevant works have been proposed in diverse areas such as computer vision, linear algebra, statistical analysis, physics and biological simulation, database analysis, computational finance and cryptography among others. The first trend on using GPUs to speed-up the execution of general purpose algorithms was somehow tricky, and involved translating algorithms into graphics terms, storing data into textures and invoking rendering operations to perform algorithm computations. In the meantime, GPU architectures have moved to a unified rendering pipeline and have included new hardware resources that can benefit the execution of different kind of applications. Programmability of GPUs has improved and new frameworks like OpenCL are available to combine the power of multi-core CPUs and GPUs in heterogeneous systems. In this chapter a complete review on GPU Computing history, techniques and principles are exposed, together with a deeper insight on the use of GPUs for computer vision and image processing applications. Finally, future trends on GPU and heterogeneous architectures programming are discussed.

Keywords: GPU Computing, GPGPU, Stream Processing

1. Introduction

The reader of this book will probably have a good understanding of the advances of computer generated graphics, as well as computer graphics technologies. It is needless to say

[*] E-mail address: marmar@tel.uva.es

that the increasing performance of the chips have been leaded by the silicon fabrication process reduction because of the needs of high performance in the primary aims of graphics hardware, rasterization and the final fragment processing.

The rasterization process is a highly independent operation performed over many 3D primitives to provide millions of fragments of an output image. The rasterization is the graphics pipeline stage where the 3D world converges to a 2D view, interpolating a variety of per-vertex descriptors such as color, texture information and normals. This interpolator has to be very powerful and optimized in order to feed the rest of the pipeline without losing an interactive framerate. Because of the independence of its operations over different memory data rasterization becomes a highly parallel task. Since the first 3D accelerator cards (apart from the video cards), this hardware stage was responsible for the most demanding floating point operations of interpolation, which was too computationally expensive for the central processing unit or CPU. Indeed, Advanced Micro Devices (AMD) proposed in 1998 an extension of the 1997 Intel single-instruction-multiple-data (SIMD) MMX technology for the AMD K6-2 microprocessors supporting floating point operations. They were called *3DNow!* as a clearly emphasized term related to 3D graphics. In 1999 Intel offered the similar SIMD technology for the Intel Pentium III processor, called *Streaming SIMD Extensions* or SSE, consisting of eight 128-bit registers and an instruction set for inherently parallel operations on regular data flows. The 3DNow!/SSE technologies were a late response for software rendering to the 3D graphics cards as they were included inside the video cards at that time.

The term GPU (Graphics Processing Unit, in contrast to the popular CPU) was coined by the manufacturer NVIDIA when its GeForce 256 card was released in 1999. The GPUs of the end of the 90's supported multitexturing capabilities and progressively increasing the number of available textures for improving realism of a 3D scenario. This hardware device was responsible for the float computation involved in rendering in a very parallel and efficient way, offloading the computational cost from the CPU. The next great revolution was the introduction of programmable stages in the graphics pipeline.

In 2001, two of the three previously fixed stages were replaced with programmable components. In this way, the hardware-accelerated programmability of GPUs was exposed to programmers for the development of specialized programs called *shaders*. These shaders could be loaded into the graphics card, replacing the fixed functionality and providing a way to customize special effects and realistic 3D scenes in real-time. However, it enabled their use to optimize general purpose computation problems and perform computational intensive algorithms. There were two kinds of shaders, called vertex and fragment shaders, and they constituted the executable code of the corresponding programmable components of the graphics pipeline. In 2002, the PhD candidate Mark Harris at the University of North Carolina at Chapel Hill used first the term GPGPU to refer to this way of general purpose computation model on GPUs, and established the well known repository `www.gpgpu.org` [31].

After some years of experimental success using these GPU platforms as vector coprocessors (or *accelerators*), the academia demanded more abstraction layers for programming them. Moreover, universities started to offer their first GPGPU courses as new ways for reaching high performance computation levels for commodity architectures. The GPU was exposed as a data-parallel computation platform that, because of its architectural design simplicity (compared to a CPU), could scale well in raw performance and transistor integration. They turned into a unified architecture very prone for general purpose data-parallel programming and the shading techniques for general programming became obsolete in some way. Graphics processors were including more and more transistors for computation purposes and they became an interesting platform for improving the efficiency of general algorithmic solutions. As a data-parallel computation platform new algorithmic reformulations were adopted in order to execute the original algorithms on this kind of computing platform, especially important for data-intensive problems such as those related to image processing, linear algebra, PDEs, etc.

On the CPU market clock frequencies were producing very high levels of consumption reaching to limits of heat dissipation. This issue has been referred to as the *power wall* and hardware architectures adopted a new design philosophy by extending the number of computational cores instead of speeding up the clock frequency of a single processor [9]. In 2004 Intel and AMD announced a new era with the multi-core as next computing platform. This tendency is now widespread and software developers need new coding styles taking in mind algorithmic reformulations in order to exploit the different cores of a commodity computer. Then, the GPU and CPU developing style converges into a natural parallel paradigm. Developing for the GPU platform is like developing for a future CPU platform with hundreds of computational cores and researchers have pushed forward a number of technical conferences around this idea [1] [33].

C for CUDA is the Nvidia proposal of a high level interface to its unified GPU hardware for general purpose computation on GPU, or *GPU Computing*. *OpenCL* is a cross-platform interface originally focused to accelerators, multicores, mobile devices, etc. At the time of writing Intel *Ct* is being planned as a new abstraction layer for Intel processors taking advantage of multi-core and vector extensions like MMX, SSE or AVX as well as their variants and future SIMD instruction sets. Intel Ct is a higher level abstraction layer than other thread-oriented libraries like OpenMP. It will focus on data-parallel approaches and safety, avoiding as much as possible indeterministic states and coding styles that could lead to race conditions and deadlocks.

Because of its importance in the recent past, present and near future, as well as its similarities to the CPU trend, this chapter introduces the *GPU Computing* area, or the use of GPUs for general-purpose computation.

2. Graphics Hardware Evolution

The need for processing and rendering 3D mathematical data on computers caused the development of multichip co-processors devoted to speed-up the inherent parallel computations behind tasks such as geometrical transformations, lighting and texturing, among others.

In 1999 NVIDIA introduced the first GPU (Graphics Processing Unit), a single chip processor based on the GeForce 256 chip, containing 23 million of transistors, and providing floating point computations at an unprecedented arithmetic throughput. In 2000 ATI Technologies launched the R100 chip-based GPUs. For 10 years NVIDIA and ATI have been tough competitors in the race of launching the fastest GPU to the day, and being the first company to fulfill the new standards functionality requirements demanded by the

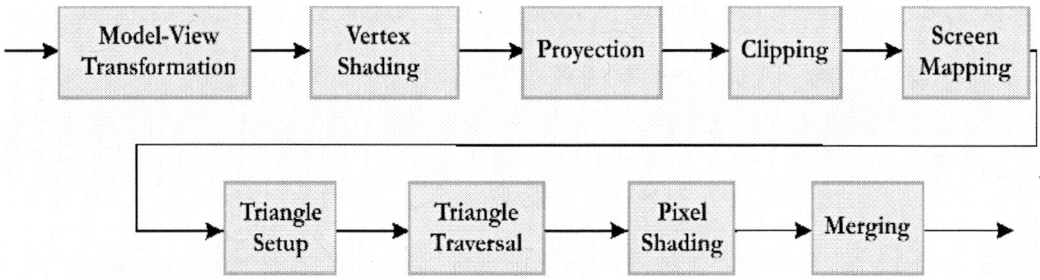

Figure 1. Fixed-function graphics pipeline.

software industry. First GPUs consisted on a not programmable, but configurable fixed-function graphics pipeline. Different stages along the pipeline were devised to different tasks, but computations inside every stage were hard-wired, thus only some parameters could be changed to obtain a different output at a given stage. Figure 1 shows a fixed-function graphics pipeline. A mathematical description of a scene is uploaded from the CPU to the GPU and a program allocated on the CPU needs a graphics API to control the GPU functionality [4].

In 2001, NVIDIA presented the Geforce 3 GPU series (based on the NV20 chip), containing the first programmable floating-point vertex stage in the graphics pipeline and native support for DirectX 8 and OpenGL extensions. Although the programmability of these GPUs was very limited and never came down to a midrange price point, they laid the foundations for further GPU generations, that would extend programmability to the pixel shader stage and make texture accessible from the vertex stage. In 2002, the ATI Radeon 9700 (based on the R300 chip) provided a programmable 24-bit floating point pixel shader processor and in 2003 the NVIDIA GeForce FX (NV30 chip) added 32-bit floating point precission [57].

In 2004 and 2005, NVIDIA launched the GeForce 6 (NV40 chip) and GeForce 7 (G70 chip) series GPUs [55]. These GPUs included separate processors dedicated to vertex and pixel processing and supported the Shader Model 3.0 functionality. The GeForce 6 Series GPUs allowed, for the first time, to fetch cached texture data from a vertex processor. Figure 2 shows a programmable graphics pipeline in which vertex, geometry and pixel processors can be programmed using shaders. Instructions inside shaders are executed in parallel over all the processing units available on the GPU. Vertex shader programs can alter the position, color or orientation of the vertices of primitives that constitute the model to be rendered onto the screen. Geometry shader programs can modify these primitives or generate new ones. Fragment or pixel shader programs can be used to compute the final or intermediate pixel color on the image at a given position. As vertices and colors can be expressed using 4-component vectors, these processors were design to perform the same operation over the different components in the same clock cycle. Also, swizzling or rearranging the elements of a vector was possible at no cost. In the graphics pipeline, between these programmable stages, there were other very fast fixed-function stages such as the rasterizer, in charged of

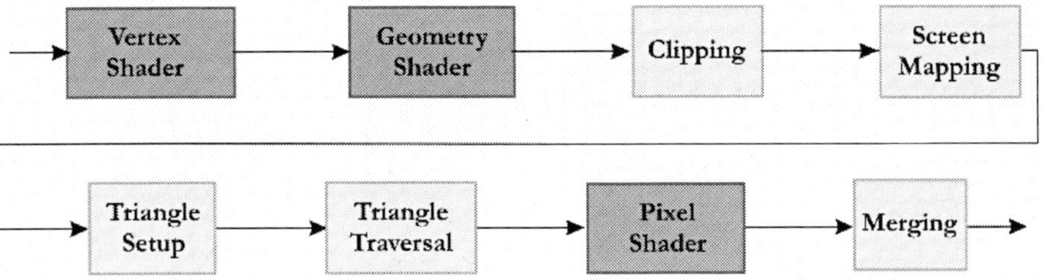

Figure 2. Programmable graphics pipeline.

generating the fragments or potential pixels laying inside a triangle.

When programmable GPUs became available, a small number of researchers had already took notice of the incredible computational performance that GPUs could provide compared to common CPUs to solve problems that could be expressed following a SIMD (Single Instruction Multiple Data) basis [23]. The figures of performance for floating point computation thrown by GPUs compared to CPUs, based on a SISD (Single Instruction Single Data), architecture already proposed by Alan Turing and Von Neumann in the 30s and 40s [109] [28], were astonishing [92]. The internal design of GPUs has evolved on a very different way than CPUs. In order to process millions of vertices and pixels in a fragment of a second, hardware parallelism has to be exploited. Most of the transistors inside a GPU die are devised to real computations, rather than cache and branching, as it happens on the CPU. The memory latency is hidden using large memory bandwidths, so that it is possible to feed a large number of processing units at once. The use of little caches is very efficient, as rendering algorithms tend to fetch data from contiguous memory locations.

However, GPUs tremendous peak power for graphics operations was not possible to achieve for non-graphics general purpose programs. First, the GPU programming model was limited by hardware constraints (i.e. scatter/gather operations were very limited and no random reads and writes could be done) [11]. In second place, GPUs had to be accessed using a graphics API such as DirectX or OpenGL and vertex and fragment shaders had to be programmed using a specific shading language such as Cg (C for graphics) or HLSL [22]. During these days, the term GPGPU (General Purpose computing on the GPU) was coined [94]. Anyone who would like to take advantage of the GPU to speed-up scientific problems had to learn the basis of the GPU architecture, new APIs and languages, how to express his problem in graphics terms and redesign the original algorithm so that it could fit on a parallel processor with lots of limitations, under programmer point of view. Although doing GPGPU was very tricky [38] [40], the results obtained were promising. More and more scientists were attracted by the possibility of performing computations faster [31] [24]. The SPMD (Single Program Multiple Data) processing model, allowed developing an application for a given GPU and get an incredible speed-up when running it on the next GPU model, which would include more and more vertex and fragment processors that could run in parallel. Figure 3 shows the architecture of a GeForce 6800 GPU. The number of fragment processors or pixel shaders in the 6 and 7 generations of NVIDIA GPUs

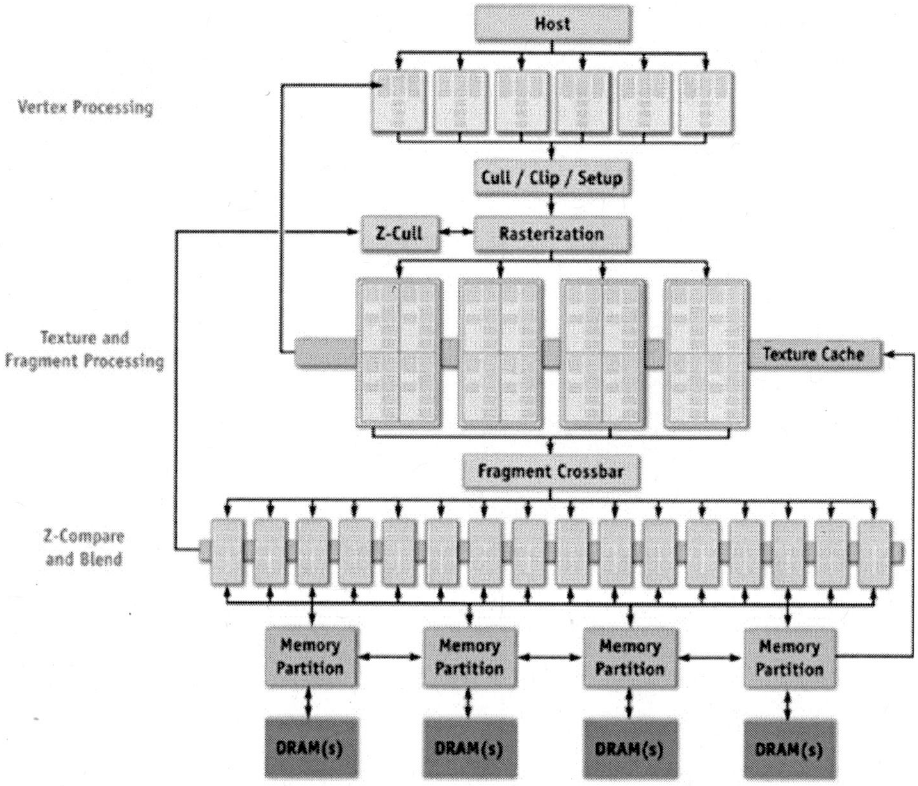

Figure 3. GeForce 6 series architecture. Vertex and fragment processing stages were performed in parallel on a varying number of separate vertex and fragment processors [55].

was considerably larger than the number of vertex processors. The GeForce 7800 GTX GPU included only 7 vertex processors, but 24 fragment processors. For this reason, using pixel shaders was the preferred choice in the first days of GPGPU. Although different stages could be programmed in the pipeline, different graphics applications need a different amount of resources in the vertex and fragment stages for maximum performance [93]. It was difficult to balance the throughput over the whole pipeline and unpredictable bottlenecks arose. For this reason, GPU designers decided to merge these stages into a unified shader architecture.

In 2006 NVIDIA launched the GeForce 8800 GPU (based on the G80 chip), in which 4-component floating point registers and processors were simplified to Scalar Processors that can operate on vertex, fragments or any other manner of data. This way, a pool of resources can be dynamically adjusted for a better load balance. Three data iterations over these scalar processors are need in case vertex, geometry and fragment operations are need. Figure 4, shows the architecture of the GeForce 8800 GTX GPU. A total of 128 scalar processors were included on it. Every scalar processor is capable of executing the code of a single thread, what results on a SIMT (Single Instruction Multiple Thread) model, in which a set of GPU Threads is executed to perform the same instruction of a kernel program, using different data, in as much scalar processors as possible. The G80-based GPUs introduced not only an important change in the GPU architectural design, but also new tools and languages to ease the programmability of GPUs for general purpose. The so called CUDA parallel computing architecture designed by NVIDIA allows programming GPUs in a high-level language such as C for CUDA or FORTRAN and map computations to further generations of GPUs that will include new hardware optimizations, guarantying the scalability of the code. NVIDIA coined the term GPU Computing for describing this new way of taking benefit of GPUs for general purpose.

A CUDA program executes pieces of code on a CPU or host and on a target GPU called device [87]. Computing pieces of code executed on the GPU are not called shaders, but kernels. Kernel instructions are executed in parallel across a set of threads called grid in CUDA terminology. These threads can do, for the first time, random writes and reads to and from global memory. The grid of threads is divided into subsets of threads called *blocks*, which are executed concurrently under a cluster of multiprocessors called Stream Multiprocessors (SM). As it is showed on Figure 4, the G80-based GPUs were designed to have up to 16 SMs, each one comprised of 8 scalar processors, for a total of 128 scalar processors on the GPU. Instructions of threads belonging to the same block of threads are executed consecutively on the same multiprocessor. The SM schedules blocks of threads in groups of 32 threads called warps and, therefore, a multiprocessor needs at least four clock cycles to process the instruction associated to 32 threads of a warp. If necessary, barrier synchronization is possible among the threads belonging to the same block, in order to guarantee that every thread in the block has reached the same execution point of the kernel. On each SM, there are 16 KB (16 banks of 1KB) of configurable on-chip cache, called shared memory in the CUDA terminology. This shared memory, is available for the programmer for data interchange among the threads of the same block of threads. Shared memory reads and writes are one order of magnitude faster than equivalent reads and writes on global memory. Also, accessing global memory under certain alignment memory patterns, allows to group memory transfers to maximize the use of memory bandwidth, under a technique known as memory coalescing. A common execution pattern in CUDA programs consist on loading a bunch of data into shared memory using every thread of a block to read 4, 8 or 16 bytes of data. A synchronization point is used to guarantee that every thread has completed the memory copy. Then, threads inside the block cooperate to perform a given operation using fast data reads and writes on shared memory. Once the result has been obtained it is written to global memory, where it can be accessed by the threads of the grid belonging to different blocks, or copied to the host system DRAM memory. During thread execution, in case a group of threads is idle due to a memory read or write, the SM can execute the instructions associated to another block of threads, hiding memory latency. As there are a limited number of resources available inside each SM (amount of registers and shared memory), this is only possible if the SM is able to allocate resources for more than one block of threads. Depending on the given application, the programmer can adjust the size of the block of threads to favor this behavior, maximizing the multiprocessor occupancy. However, a larger occupancy do not necessarily result in a greater performance [86].

In 2008 NVIDIA presented a revision of the previous core G80, the GT200. The number of transistors in this architecture was risen from 681M to 1400M. The first GPUs which included this new chip were the GeForce GTX 280, the Quadro FX5800 and the 10-series family of Tesla GPUs. The latter oriented exclusively to the GPU Computing market and lacking VGA or DVI connectors. These new GPUs included more registers and the number of scalar processors was raised to 240 (see Table 1). Up to 30 SMs are available on the GPUs

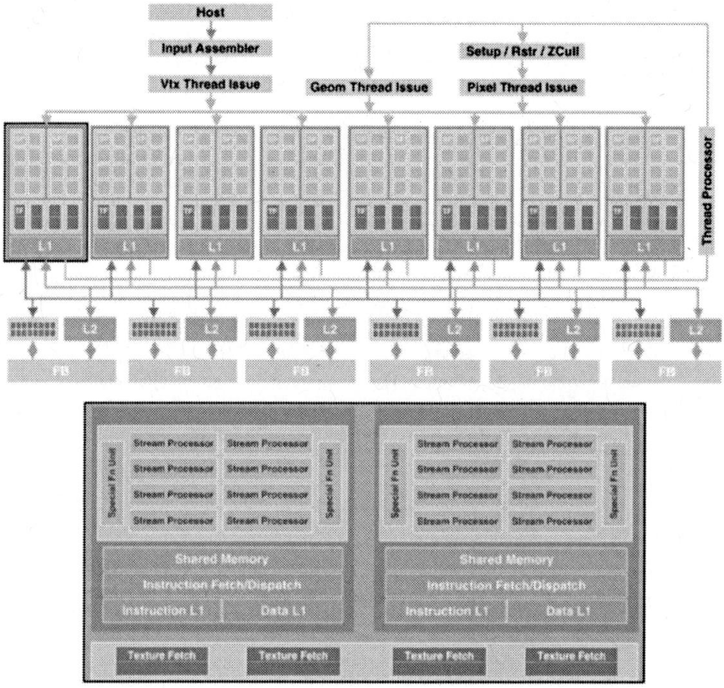

Figure 4. GeForce 8800 GTX GPU unified architecture [93].

based on the G80 core. Some improvements were made so that memory coalescing could be speeded-up in hardware. Also, although not as fast as floating-point computations, double precision computations, very important in many scientific fields, were finally possible on these new GPUs.

In September 2009, during the GPU Technology Conference [33], NVIDIA announced a new graphics architecture, one step further for GPU Computing. The new chip architecture GF100 -codenamed Fermi-, heavily emphasis on general computing, and an effort has been made so that the new GPUs are adequate for professional HPC (High Performance Computing) clusters, i.e. including ECC support. This feature prevents soft-error bit changes caused by the natural radiation to which large hardware installations are subject to. Fermi chips are the first GPUs to have a real cache hierarchy, with Level 1 caches to keep specific information on hand and a single, shared Level 2 cache for larger tasks. They also provide faster context switching and graphics interoperability. In March 2010, the first Fermi-based GPUs, the GeForce GTX 480 and the GeForce GTX 470, were made available. The GF100 based GPUs introduce an important leap over the previous GT200 based GPUs, in terms of architectural design and transistor count. A total of 3200 million transistors are used on the GF100 die. A 384-bit memory interface can access 6 x 64 bit memory partitions and up to 6 GB of GDDR5 DRAM are allowed.

Figure 5 shows the architecture of GF100 based GPUs. Traditionally, GPUs had been designed maximizing the number of transistors in the silicon to perform operations, rather

Table 1. Comparison table of the latest NVIDIA GPU chips.

GPU	G80	GT200	Fermi
Transistors	681 million	1.4 billion	3.0 billion
CUDA Cores	128	240	512
Double Precision Floating Point Capability	None	30 FMA ops/clock	256 FMA ops/clock
Single Precision Floating Point Capability	128 MAD ops/clock	240 MAD ops/clock	512 FMA ops/clock
Special Function Units (SFUs)/ SM	2	2	4
Warp schedulers (per SM)	1	1	2
Shared Memory (per SM)	16 KB	16 KB	Configurable 48 KB or 16 KB
L1 Cache (per SM)	None	None	Configurable 16 KB or 48 KB
L2 Cache	None	None	768 KB
ECC Memory Support	No	No	Yes
Concurrent Kernels	No	No	Up to 16
Load/Store Address Width	32-bit	32-bit	64-bit

than cache or branching. GPU programs have enough parallelism and hide memory latency. However, this is not true for any general purpose program. In an effort to provide a more flexible architecture, Fermi GPUs have configurable on-chip shared memory and L1 cache. From 16 KB (G80 and GT200) to 64 KB, that can be configured as 48KB/16KB of shared memory and L1 cache, respectively, or vice versa. Applications not using shared memory take benefit automatically from the L1 cache. Applications with lots of memory accesses (low arithmetic intensity) that are bandwidth constrained take benefit of more shared memory resources (more blocks can be launched). Up to 16 SMs are available to perform computations, but now each one is filled with 32 scalar processors (4x the number of processors in GT200), for a total of 512 scalar processors in one GPU. The third generation of SMs add many new features. The double precision peak performance has increased by an 8x factor and up to 16 double precision fused multiply-add (FMA) operations per clock can be performed on each SM. Inside every scalar processor, an integer ALU of 32 bits precision (GT200 provided 24 bits) and a floating point unit FPU can be found. The FPU provides FMA instructions for both single and double precision arithmetic. Also, special function units (SFUs) execute transcendental instructions such as sin, cosine, reciprocal, and square root. In Fermi GPUs each SM has two warp schedulers so that instructions from two different warps can be executed concurrently. This execution model avoids idle threads hiding memory latency, but is only possible when double precision is not needed. On the GT200 based GPUs, different kernels of the same program had to be executed serially. The GPU hardware resources were delivered to the threads conforming the grid launched at the kernel call. In the Fermi architecture, each SM is able to execute blocks of threads belonging to different grids, opening the door to task parallelism inside the same GPU.

3. GPU Programming for General Purpose

The introduction of the first programmable GPUs, caused researchers all around the world started to explore the possibility of using these parallel processors to solve scientific and engineering problems in a faster way. In the first times of GPGPU, programmability of

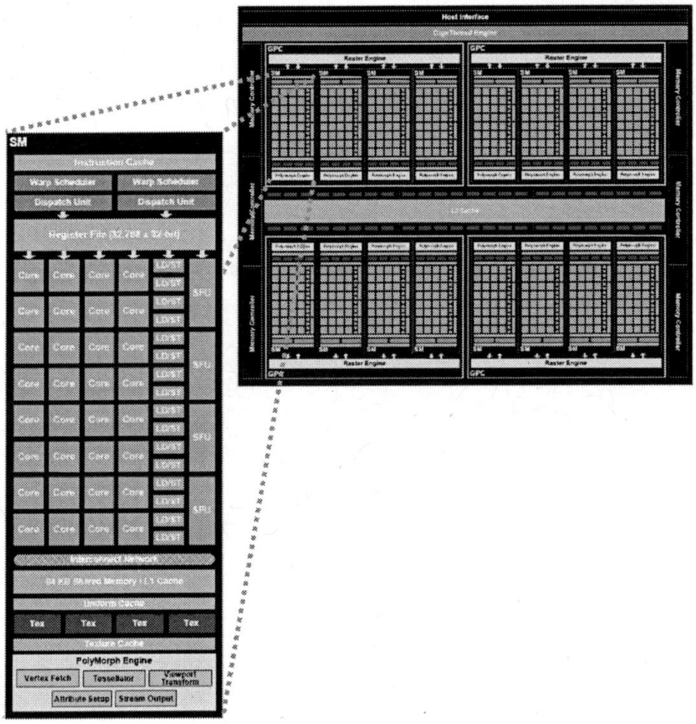

Figure 5. The GF100 chip (codename Fermi). First GPU designed for massively parallel computing.

GPUs for general purpose was done using a graphics API and a shading language, thus was a hard task for developers who were not experts at computer graphics. However, the interest on using the GPU as an accelerator, encouraged many scientists to learn at least the basis of the OpenGL/DirectX graphics APIs and Cg/HLSL shading languages, and also study the principles of design under the GPU architecture. A few years after, hundreds of research papers were available and GPU manufacturers had designed new hardware and software platforms to ease the utilization of GPUs for general purpose computing. Today, the new trend known as *GPU Computing* has taken over the old GPGPU school for programming the GPU. The aim of this section is to briefly compare both approaches.

3.1. GPGPU: General Purpose computing on the GPU

Traditionally, accessing the GPU computational resources involved translating the problem into native graphics operations. Computation takes place through graphics APIs calls, which are used to upload initial data from the CPU to GPU textures; and shading languages, which are used to execute a fragment or vertex program under the data allocated in parallel, using a SPMD *(Single Program Multiple Data)* model. First GPUs presented certain restrictions for memory writing operations. The output of a fragment shader is rendered to a given position in the *framebuffer*, that has been established already before the execution of the program. On the other hand, accessing arbitrary data from a fragment program is not only possible, but convenient. In case several data has to be read from a fragment program in a neighborhood of one or more textures, a cached 2D access is done, what makes GPUs very convenient for certain computer graphics operations such as image filtering. The result of the fragment program can be rendered to an output texture that can be used again as data input in the entrance of the graphics pipeline. In general, a simple GPGPU application is divided in the next steps:

1. The programmer specifies a geometric primitive that covers the computational domain of interest. A typical geometric primitive is a rectangle or *quad*, which covers exactly the size of a texture containing float values. This matrix contains data previously uploaded from the CPU. An orthogonal projection is selected and the rasterizer generates a fragment for every pixel under this geometry.

2. A fragment program is executed then over each one of the generated fragments. The same program is executed in parallel in as many as fragment processors are available in the GPU under a SPMD (Single Program Multiple Data). The texture coordinates of input data have been interpolated by the rasterizer, so that inside the fragment program it is possible to access one or more data elements in the input texture.

3. The fragment program is used to do some mathematical operations over the data allocated in the input texture and gathered using texture operations. It is possible to read not only from just one, but several input textures. In case these textures are of type LUMINANCE a single float value can be stored by texel, but in case RGBA textures are used, up to four-component vectors can be uploaded by texel. Shading languages incorporate mathematical operations that can be performed simultaneously over these four-component vectors.

4. The result of the fragment program is rendered to the *framebuffer*, or, alternatively, to an output texture of the same or different dimensions of the initial computational domain. This texture can be then used for further computations. Also, multiple render target support allows to generate different outputs onto different textures from the same fragment processor.

Therefore, programming the GPU under the old GPGPU point of view, requires using the graphics hardware in a much similar way as any graphics application. The terminology used for the development of these applications is very different to the one used for developing general purpose applications. For this reason, some authors proposed to study the graphics hardware as a *stream processor* [38].

3.2. GPU Computing

As stated before, one of the main restrictions of traditional GPGPU techniques was the necessity to translate data computations to graphics terms, although the final applications has nothing to do with graphics. New high level languages such as C for CUDA or OpenCL, solve this problem providing more generic interfaces, that allow the programmer a more immediate and adequate access to the hardware resources. An application using these interfaces is organized as follows:

1. The programmer defines the domain of computation as a *grid of threads*. Each thread will be in charged of processing one or more parts of the computational domain. Threads are grouped in *blocks of threads* which can share data among them and synchronize.

2. A *kernel* function defines the code that would be executed by the grid of threads in parallel in a SIMT (Single Instruction Multiple Data) fashion. The programming model is more flexible, as different threads can perform different operations. Different blocks of threads are assigned to different multiprocessors.

3. Every thread can perform mathematical and memory access operations. In contrast to shading languages, mathematical operations are designed for scalar values. Also, the same input buffer can be used to store the final output and random writes are allowed.

4. The final buffer can be used as input to another kernel function. Newer architectures such as Fermi based GPUs allow to execute in parallel different kernels on the same GPU.

Although CUDA and OpenCL interfaces do not require the utilization of graphics APIs, they have methods for graphics interoperability. This way, not only general purpose applications, but also traditional graphics applications can take benefit of these new processing models and the underlying hardware resources.

4. Computational Primitives on the GPU

Developing general purpose applications on the GPU require adapting one or more basic operations, or computational primitives, for our own requirements. In this section, the main computational primitives: scatter/gather, map, reduction and scan are described.

4.1. Map

Map is one of the basic operations in the context of parallelism. It consists on applying the same function (*kernel*) over a collection of data elements (*stream*). A serial implementation would consist on a loop that iteratively executes the function over the elements in the stream. Execution time of this kind of operations can be reduced considerably if each operation inside the function is performed simultaneously over some elements of the stream. On a classic GPGPU application, data in the stream is stored on a texture, and a fragment shader is applied in parallel over as much fragments as fragment processors are available in the GPU. Typically, one fragment is processed to compute a single result that is stored on a texel on an output texture. In the newer GPU Computing high level interfaces such as CUDA or OpenCL, the code to be executed in parallel is indeed called *kernel*. The kernel is executed in a SIMT *(Single Instruction Multiple Thread)* fashion, and thousands of GPU treads can be launched simultaneously, each one operating on their own data. Threads can randomly read and write from any position in global memory, although some restrictions can be applied to read and write from consecutive positions, so that reads and writes are grouped into a small number of memory transfers, maximizing memory bandwidth utilization.

4.2. Scatter and gather

The terms scatter and gather are referred to the possibility of writing or reading in arbitrary positions of memory. A scatter operation in C language can be expressed as $hvector[i] = data$, where the value $data$ is stored in the position indexed as i on the data vector $hvector$. On the other hand, a gather operation is employed for reading arbitrary data, in C language the expression $data = hvector[i]$ is used to read the value stored in the component indexed as i in vector $hvector$ to the scalar variable $data$. From the classic GPGPU point of view, textures can be used to perform arbitrary reading operations (gather) inside fragment programs, where data indexing is done using texture coordinates. However, scatter operations over textures are more complex, since every fragment output is associated to a given position on the frame buffer, or on the texture to which the result is rendered to. There are different techniques to get around this limitation [11]. One of the most common techniques consists on using vertex programs. In vertex programs, it is possible to specify the final position for the vertex, thus the final position of the result on the texture. Luckily, new hardware, APIs and interfaces such as CUDA have improved programmability for scatter and gather operations. Arrays, pointers and variables can now be used in the same manner as in a general purpose language like C.

4.3. Reduction

Many general purpose applications require performing a global computation in which the value of every single element in a collection of data is considered. That is, for example, summing-up the value of every element, computing the average value, the minimum or the maximum, among many other possible operations. Usually, for this global computations, a collection of input data (input stream) turns into a collection of output data (output stream) that is smaller. In the previous examples, the output will actually be a single scalar value. In the GPGPU old school, reductions were performed rendering intermediate results onto textures. The final result is obtained after a series of shader passes along the graphics pipeline. In the simplest case of using a unidimensional texture to store the input stream, a fragment program is used to read two consecutive values and render the result of an operation between both elements (summation, average, minimum,...) on a texel in an output texture. This output texture is used as the input texture in the next shader pass, in a technique known as *ping-pong*. On each iteration, the computational domain is reduced to a half, upon the first texel in one of the textures used in the ping-pong has the final result of the reduction operation in its first texel. In case of using bidimensional textures, four different input texels can be read in each fragment, so that in each iteration the computational domain is reduced to one fourth of its size. Figure 6 illustrates the steps of a reduction operation to compute the maximum value over the elements stored on a bidimensional texture. For bidimensional reductions less shader passes are necessary to obtain the final result. Also, GPUs have small texture caches, optimized for 2D data locality. For this reason, reductions using bidimensional textures are very fast. On the other hand, reductions can be performed using CUDA and OpenCL interfaces. In these cases, a group of threads cooperate in the same manner as a group of fragment processors do, to obtain intermediate results of the reduction to which it is possible to apply the same algorithm several times to obtain the final result.

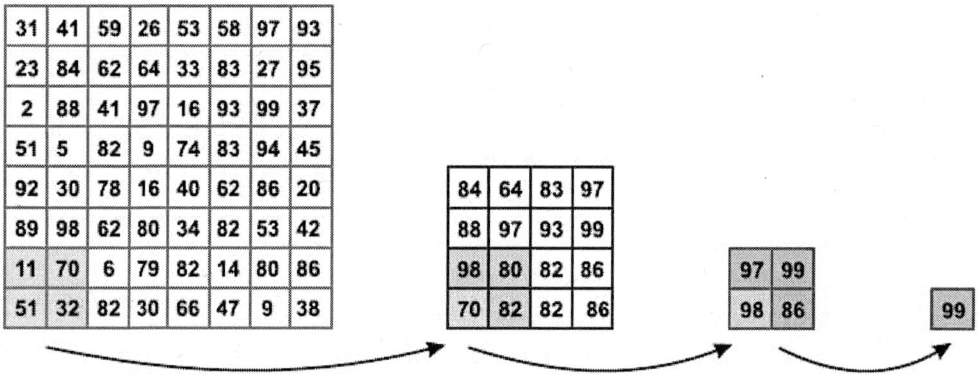

Figure 6. Bidimensional reduction. On each shader pass a reduction (in the example max operation) is performed over groups of four values, thus the size computational domain is divided by four.

4.4. Scan

Scan primitive is very useful in many algorithms in which parallel computation can be applied [43]. For a given collection A of data elements, the scan operation returns a collection B of data elements of the same length, in which each element $B[i]$ stores the result of computing a summing-up reduction of the previous elements in A, $B[i] = \sum_{j=0}^{j=i-1} A[j]$. Blelloch describes a large variety of potential applications of scan, from sorting methods such as quicksort to sparse matrix operations [7]. The first implementation of scan in GPU was presented by Horn and applied to collision detection and adaptive subdivision surface tessellation [49]. Hensley et al. employed a similar implementation for integral image computation on the GPU [42]. The Horn and Hensley algorithms present a complexity $O(n \log_2 n)$, a factor $\log_2 n$ worst than the optimal sequential solution. Sengupta et al. [100] and Gress et al. [32] presented implementations with complexity $O(n)$. Gress proposed the use of the GPU for the detection of collisions of deformable parametrized surfaces, building a list of pairs of bounding boxes and using a scan operation to delete those pairs that do not intersect. Sengupta breaks this method into two stages: a reduction step and a collecting stage to take full benefit of the parallelism provided by the GPU. All these methods were programmed with the old GPGPU techniques, using a graphics API and a shading language. Harris et al. [39] presented an efficient implementation of the scan algorithm using CUDA. In their implementation, the performance is up to $\times 7$ times faster than the GPGPU version and takes benefit from shared memory and advanced techniques such as loop unrolling. As a result of this work, the library CUDPP (CUDA Data Parallel Primitives) turns up [85]. This library offers the programmer a collection of computational primitives such as reductions, sorting, scan or random number generation, that can be used to build more complex CUDA applications.

5. Fields of interest

Since the aparition of the programmable stages in graphics processors, researchers all around the world found a field to explore the migration of their algorithms for their execution under a low-cost, but high-performance parallel architecture. Works related to linear algebra [62, 29, 80, 25] and physical process simulation [36, 37, 69, 56, 114], image processing [45, 112, 16, 103] and computer vision [113, 111, 67, 104] are pioneers in the use of GPUs for general purpose computing. The introduction of a unified shading architecture and high-level interfaces such as CUDA, have allowed in the last years to extend the use of the GPU to a larger range of problems [84].

5.1. Linear Algebra

Linear algebra is one of the fields that more attention has received [62, 107, 35, 59]. Matrix-based algebra computations are the building blocks of several algorithms and applications such as PDE resolution. A representative work is the one proposed by Krüger y Westermann, which proposes sparse vector and matrix computations on the GPU for fluid simulation using the Navier-Stokes approach. Other remarkable works are those presented by Fatahalian et al. [21] for dense matrix multiplication and Galoppo et al.[25] in which the GPU is used to solve dense linear systems. The performance obtained on the GPU is higher than using optimized ATLAS implementations on the CPU. The availability of high-level interfaces such as CUDA has simplified and enhanced linear algebra related operations in the GPU. Nvidia provides CUBLAS [17], a library implemented in *C for CUDA* that follows the popular BLAS (*Basic Linear Algebra Subprograms*) convention.

An immediate application of matrix representation and operation under the GPUs is the resolution of ordinary differential equations (ODEs) and partial differential equations (PDEs) [8] [63]. For PDE resolution finite-differences methods and finite-elements methods (FEM) can be used and traditionally the first have been more used on the GPU [90]. One of the first works for PDEs resolution using a graphics API is the one presented by Rumpf y Strzodka [98, 97]. Goeddeke et al. showed also the convenience of the GPU for PDE resolution [27]. In that moment, double precision support on the GPU was not available, and they proposed a mixed correction in CPU-GPU that resulted $\times 2$ times faster than a CPU version.

Also, motivated by the high arithmetic capability of the GPU, several projects have developed GPU implementations of the Fast Fourier Transformation (FFT) [76, 81, 110, 10, 53, 99, 105]. In general, these implementations can use 1D and 2D input data. The library *libgpufft*, developed by Horns [48, 91] is one of the first attempts to provide a FFT based GPU code block for the developing of general purpose programs. Nowadays, Nvidia provides a simple interface for FFT computation (CUFFT) under CUDA compatible architectures [18]. This library supports double precision and up to 3D input data.

GPUs have been also used for sorting and searching operations under large collections of data. In the literature, it is possible to find adapted methods for binary search [47] or nearest neighbour search [12]. Govindaraju et al. describe in [30] an algorithm called *GPUTeraSort* for large data collection sorting. The algorithm is used to sort databases containing thousands of millions of keys.

5.2. Image Processing and Computer Vision

The SIMD (Single Instruction Multiple Data) model, in which each element has to be independent from the rest, is perfect for vertex and fragment processing, thus very convenient for many tasks related to image processing or computer vision, where it is common that operations have to be done independently over single pixels or over a neighborhood of pixels. One of the first works in which the GPU was used for image processing was developed by Yang et al. [112]. In their work they compare the SIMD capabilities of the CPUs (through MMX instructions from Intel) and the computational power of the GPUs. Using a GPU GeForce 4 an improvement of 30% is achieved with respect to a CPU Pentium 4 2.2GHz for smoothing and segmentation operations based in morphology-based operations. Segmentation techniques based on surface deformation have been also successfully adapted to the GPU computation model [97, 63, 65, 64, 101]. More recently, works using the graphics hardware to accelerate variational methods have been presented. These have been applied to tasks related to image registration, region correspondence in stereo vision, noise reducing and segmentation [106, 72].

The methods for graph partitioning have been applied in several problems in artificial vision. One of the first works that propose their adaptation for GPU was the one presented by Dixit et al. [19]. As it is showed in [50, 108, 26], the use of global and shared memory in CUDA and the possibility of performing atomic operations has allowed to improve the performance of these methods. Strozdka and Garbe presented a method for movement estimation through eigenvectors analysis [103]. For video compression, Kelly and Kokaram [54] describe a movement estimator based that uses a hierarchical algorithm robust to noise. Mizukami et al. present in [77] an implementation of the regularization method proposed by Horn and Schunk [46], together with a multiscale search for optical flow computation. Dumortier et al. [20] present a library adapting the Lukas-Kanade method for optic flow computation on CUDA architectures, reporting an speedup of $\times 55$. In [41], a method for processing video at 640×480 px resolution and 90 fps using a GeForce 8800 GTX and four different scales, is presented. An equivalent implementation in CPU (Pentium 4 3 GHz) for images at resolution 320×240 and only 3 levels of scale, works only at 1 fps.

Many works related to 2D and 3D tracking on the GPU use the particle filter as a framework for solving visual tracking problems [78, 79, 95, 61, 58, 70, 66, 82]. This method require the evaluation of multiple independent hypothesis, thus it is a clear candidate for a parallel implementation [13]. Other approaches, as the one proposed in [68] use an adaptation of the Mean Shift algorithm.

For pattern recognition, several researchers have shown great results in means of performance with their GPU-based artificial neural network implementations, speeding up execution dozens of times [96, 89, 102, 71, 14, 6, 83, 74, 73]. Tze-Yui Ho et al. [44], explains the advantages and disadvantages of using a GPU-based simulation of a cellular neural network (CNN) instead of other methods such as VLSI circuits. The results show that the GPU-based CNN simulator can run $\times 8-17$ times faster than a CPU-based CNN simulator, improving the performance at a low cost. Just as in other research fields, newer proposals map existing algorithms to the CUDA stream processing model [60, 75]. Honghoon Jang et al. [52] designed a heterogeneous implementation for pattern recognition and image processing, using CUDA for execution on the GPU, and OpenMP for execution on a multi-core

CPU. For text detection, the hybrid implementation performed about $\times 15$ times faster than an implementation using only the CPU and about $\times 4$ times faster than an implementation using only the GPU.

5.3. Conferences and Workshops

The first international workshop associated with the idea of using graphics hardware for general-purpose computation was held in Los Angeles in 2004 as GP^2 (General-Purpose Computation on Graphics Processors) [3]. It was scheduled some days before ACM SIGGRAPH 2004, the first large conference to offer a full day tutorial on GPGPU techniques. Next year, and even in the infancy of the topic, the ACM SIGGRAPH 2005 offered again a full day tutorial on GPGPU techniques as a nice indication of the relevance of its potential with the preliminary appearance of the Rapidmind seed (later Intel Ct) or the origins of CUDA. Since the GP^2 many workshops and conferences have grown showing promising applications of GPU Computing as stand-alone conferences [5, 2] or workshops in conjunction with other conferences [51, 1, 15]. However, the explosion of dedicated conferences came in 2008-2009 with a more general adoption of higher level languages like C for CUDA. The GPU Technology Conference (formerly Nvision conference) [88, 33, 34] is the Nvidia showcase for releasing their latest news, but also a nice forum around GPU Computing, with tutorials on OpenCL, CUDA, DirectCompute, new technologies, keynote speakers and hundreds of applications. A list of some past conferences can be found in the reference section.

6. Conclusion

Computer architecture is evolving fast, its trend is moving forward from a single and fast execution unit with large memory space to several execution units with small local memory. Nowadays, multi-core processors are common consumer systems. They are progressively replacing high energy-consumption desktop computers with great success and performance gains and the industry predicts that future computing systems will benefit from this scalable technology. This evolution is highly beneficial for data-parallel programs, where independent data processing takes place in the algorithms. An example of a future platform is the massively parallel graphics processing unit (GPU), with lots of execution units, small and fast memory for each processing core and high memory bandwidth. Using this platform for demonstration purposes, we can test algorithmic approaches that would scale well to new generations of desktop computers. Massively parallel architectures have arrived and developers have to made an effort to devise new algorithmic approaches, mainly in fields that require computational demanding tasks, in order to adapt them to new and future platforms.

Is the GPU platform a mainstream computing one? Probably not yet. Some authors manifest inconveniences of programming the GPU as a mainstream platform. Although huge advances since the original GPGPU *printf*-debugging style it is still a challenge. However, the Nvidia Fermi architecture is a set forward in the right direction. The PCI Express link is still a bottleneck in some applications, so direct input and output facilities are some desirable properties. The convergence between the familiar multi-core CPU and the vector co-processor, that the GPU seems to be now, will probably become the next move for the future computing platform.

References

[1] *General-Purpose GPU Computing: Practice And Experience*, Tampa, Florida, 1983.

[2] *Workshop on GPU Supercomputing*, National Taiwan University, Taipei, 2009. Center for Quantum Science and Engineering.

[3] ACM. *ACM Workshop on General-Purpose Computation on Graphics Processors (GP2)*, 2004. Co-located with ACM SIGGRAPH.

[4] Tomas Akenine-Möller, Eric Haines, and Natty Hoffman. *Real-Time Rendering 3rd Edition.* A. K. Peters, Ltd., Natick, MA, USA, 2008.

[5] *General Purpose Computation on GPUs in Astronomy and Astrophysics (AstroGPU 2007)*, Princeton, NJ, 2007. Institute for Advanced Study.

[6] Fabrice Bernhard and Renaud Keriven. Spiking neurons on gpus. In Vassil N. Alexandrov, Geert Dick van Albada, Peter M.A. Sloot, and Jack Dongarra, editors, *Computational Science – ICCS 2006*, volume 3994 of *LNCS*, pages 236–243. Springer, 2006.

[7] Guy E. Blelloch. *Vector Models for Data-Parallel Computing*. MIT Press, 1990.

[8] J. Bolz, I. Farmer, E. Grinspun, and P. Schröoder. Sparse matrix solvers on the GPU: conjugate gradients and multigrid. *ACM Trans. Graph.*, 22(3):917–924, 2003.

[9] Andre R. Brodtkorb, Christopher Dyken, Trond R. Hagen, Jon M. Hjelmervik, and Olaf O. Storaasli. State-of-the-art in heterogeneous computing. *Sci. Program.*, 18(1):1–33, 2010.

[10] I. Buck, T. Foley, D. Horn, J. Sugerman, K. Fatahalian, M. Houston, and P. Hanrahan. Brook for GPUs: Stream computing on graphics hardware. *ACM Trans. Graph.*, 23(3):777–786, 2004.

[11] Ian Buck. Gpu computation strategies and tips. In Matt Pharr, editor, *GPU Gems 2*, chapter 32, pages 509–519. Addison Wesley, March 2005.

[12] B. Bustos, O. Deussen, S. Hiller, and D. Keim. A graphics hardware accelerated algorithm for nearest neighbor search. In *Proceedings of the 6th Int. Conf. Comput. Sci. Lecture Notes in Computer vol. 3994*, 2006.

[13] Raúl Cabido, Antonio S. Montemayor, Juan José; Pantrigo, and Bryson R. Payne. Multiscale and local search methods for real time region tracking with particle filters: local search driven by adaptive scale estimation on gpus. *Mach. Vision Appl.*, 21(1):43–58, 2009.

[14] Alexander Campbell, Erik Berglund, and Alexander Streit. Graphics hardware implementation of the parameter-less self-organising map. In Marcus Gallagher, James M. Hogan, and Frédéric Maire, editors, *IDEAL*, volume 3578 of *Lecture Notes in Computer Science*, pages 343–350. Springer, 2005.

[15] *First Computational Intelligence on Consumer Games and Graphics Hardware (CIGPU 2008)*, Hong Kong, 2008. In conjunction with IEEE World Congress on Computational Intelligence Conference (WCCI).

[16] P. Colantoni, N. Boukala, and J. D. Rugna. Fast and accurate color image processing uusing 3D graphics cards. In *Proceedings of Vision, Modeling and Visualization 2002*, 2003.

[17] The CUBLAS Library. Technical report, NVIDIA, 2009.

[18] The CUFFT Library. Technical report, NVIDIA, 2009.

[19] N. Dixit, R. Keriven, and N. Paragios. Gpu-cuts: Combinatorial optimisation, graphic processing units and adaptive object extraction. Technical report, Technical report, CERTIS, 2005.

[20] Y. Dumortier and J. Marzat. Lucas and Kanade optical flow algorithm using CUDA (LKCUDA). http://www.nvidia.com/object/cuda_home.html, 2008.

[21] K. Fatahalian, J. Sugerman, and P. Hanrahan. Understanding the efficiency of GPU algorithms for matrix-matrix multiplication. In *Proceedings of Graphics Hardware 2004*, 2004.

[22] Randima Fernando and Mark J. Kilgard. *The Cg Tutorial: The Definitive Guide to Programmable Real-Time Graphics*. Addison-Wesley Longman Publishing Co., Inc., Boston, MA, USA, 2003.

[23] M. Flynn. Some computer organizations and their effectiveness. *IEEE Trans. Comput.*, C-21:948+, 1972.

[24] James Fung and Steve Mann. Computer vision signal processing on graphics processing units. In *Proceedings of the IEEE International Conference on Acoustics, Speech, and Signal Processing (ICASSP 2004)*, volume 1, pages V–93 – V–96, Montreal, Quebec, Canada, May 2004.

[25] N. Galoppo, N. K. Govindaraju, M. Henson, and D. Manocha. LU-GPU: Efficient Algorithms for Solving Dense Linear Systems on Graphics Hardware. In *Proceedings of the 2005 ACM/IEEE conference on Supercomputing (SC '05)*, page 3, Washington, DC, USA, 2005. IEEE Computer Society.

[26] Z. A. Garrett and H. Saito. Real-Time Online Video Object Silhouette Extraction Using Graph Cuts on the GPU. In *Proceedings of the 15th International Conference on Image Analysis and Processing (ICIAP '09)*, pages 985–994, Berlin, Heidelberg, 2009. Springer-Verlag.

[27] D. Göddeke, R. Strzodka, and S. Turek. Accelerating Double Precision FEM Simulations with GPUs. In *Proceedings of the 18th Symposium on Simulation Technique*, 2005.

[28] M. D. Godfrey and D. F. Hendry. The computer as von neumann planned it. *IEEE Ann. Hist. Comput.*, 15(1):11–21, 1993.

[29] N. Goodnight, C. Woolley, G. Lewin, D. Luebke, and G. Humphreys. A multigrid solver for boundary value problems using programmable graphics hardware. In *Proceedings of the ACM SIGGRAPH/EUROGRAPHICS conference on Graphics hardware (HWWS '03)*, pages 102–111, Aire-la-Ville, Switzerland, Switzerland, 2003. Eurographics Association.

[30] N. K. Govindaraju, J. Gray, R. Kumar, and D. Manocha. GPUTeraSort: High performance graphics coprocessor sorting for large database management. In *Proceedings of the 2006 ACM SIGMOD International Conference onManagement of Data*, 2006.

[31] GPGPU: General-purpose computation using graphics hardware. `http://www.gpgpu.org`, 2010.

[32] Alexander Greß, Michael Guthe, and Reinhard Klein. Gpu-based collision detection for deformable parameterized surfaces. *Comput. Graph. Forum*, 25(3):497–506, 2006.

[33] *GPU Technology Conference 2009 (GTC)*, San José, CA, 2009.

[34] *GPU Technology Conference 2010 (GTC)*, San José, CA, 2009.

[35] J. D. Hall, N. A. Carr, and J. C. Hart. Cache and Bandwidth Aware Matrix Multiplication on the GPU. Technical report, University of Illinois, 2003.

[36] M. J. Harris, G. Coombe, T. Scheuermann, and A. Lastra. Physically-based visual simulation on graphics hardware. In *Proceedings of the ACM SIGGRAPH/EUROGRAPHICS conference on Graphics hardware (HWWS '02)*, pages 109–118, Aire-la-Ville, Switzerland, Switzerland, 2002. Eurographics Association.

[37] M. J. Harris, W. Baxter III, T. Scheuermann, and A. Lastra. Simulation of Cloud Dynamics on Graphics Hardware. In *ACM SIGGRAPH 2005 Courses (SIGGRAPH '05)*, 2003.

[38] Mark Harris. Mapping computational concepts to gpus. In Matt Pharr, editor, *GPU Gems 2*, chapter 31, pages 493–508. Addison Wesley, 2005.

[39] Mark Harris. Parallel prefix sum (scan) with cuda. In Hubert Nguyen, editor, *GPU Gems 3*, chapter 39, pages 851–876. Addison Wesley Professional, 2007.

[40] Mark Harris and Ian Buck. Gpu flow control idioms. In Matt Pharr, editor, *GPU Gems 2*, chapter 34, pages 547–555. Addison Wesley, March 2005.

[41] D. C. Hauagge. Optical Flow Algorithm using CUDA and OpenCV. http://www.liv.ic.unicamp.br/~hauagge/Daniel_Cabrini_Hauagge/Home_Page_files/CUDABOF.zip, 2008.

[42] Justin Hensley, Thorsten Scheuermann, Greg Coombe, Montek Singh, and Anselmo Lastra. Fast summed-area table generation and its applications. *Comput. Graph. Forum*, 24(3):547–555, 2005.

[43] W. Daniel Hillis and Guy L. Steele Jr. Data parallel algorithms. *Commun. ACM*, 29(12):1170–1183, 1986.

[44] Tze-Yui Ho, Anjin Park, and Keechul Jung. Parallelization of cellular neural networks on gpu. *Pattern Recogn.*, 41(8):2684–2692, 2008.

[45] M. Hopf and T. Ertl. Accelerating Morphological Analysis with Graphics Hardware. In *Proceedings of the Workshop on Vision, Modelling, and Visualization (VMV '00)* , pages 337–345. infix, 2000.

[46] B. Horn and B. Schunck. Determining optical flow. *Artificical Intelligence*, 17:185–203, 1981.

[47] D. Horn. *GPU Gems 2: Programming Techniques for High-Performance Graphics and General-Purpose Computation*, chapter 36 Stream Reduction Operations for GPGPU Applications. Addison Wesley, 2005.

[48] D. Horn. libgpufft. http://sourceforge.net/projects/gpufft/, 2006.

[49] Daniel Horn. Stream reduction operations. In Matt Pharr, editor, *GPU Gems 2*, chapter 36, pages 573–587. Addison Wesley, March 2005.

[50] M. Hussein, A. Varshney, , and L. Davis. On implementing graph cuts on cuda. In *Proceedings of the First Workshop on General Purpose Processing on Graphics Processing Units*, 2007.

[51] *GPGPU Workshop: Methods, Algorithms and Applications* , Reading, UK, 2006.

[52] Honghoon Jang, Anjin Park, and Keechul Jung. Neural network implementation using cuda and openmp. In *DICTA '08: Proceedings of the 2008 Digital Image Computing: Techniques and Applications*, pages 155–161, Washington, DC, USA, 2008. IEEE Computer Society.

[53] T. Jansen, B. Von Rymon-Lipinski, N. Hanssen, and E. Keeve. Fourier volume rendering on the GPU using a SplitStreamFFT. In *Proceedings of Vision, Modeling, and Visualization*, 2004.

[54] F. Kelly and A. Kokaram. Graphics hardware for gradient based motion estimation. *Embedded Processors for Multimedia and Communications* , 5309:92–103, 2004.

[55] Emmett Kilgariff and Randima Fernando. The geforce 6 series gpu architecture. In Matt Pharr, editor, *GPU Gems 2*, chapter 30, pages 471–491. Addison Wesley, 2005.

[56] T. Kim and M. C Lin. Visual simulation of ice crystal growth. In *Proceedings of the 2003 ACM SIGGRAPH/Eurographics symposium on Computer animation (SCA '03)*, pages 86–97, Aire-la-Ville, Switzerland, Switzerland, 2003. Eurographics Association.

[57] David B. Kirk and Wen-mei W. Hwu. *Programming Massively Parallel Processors: A Hands-on Approach*. Morgan Kaufmann, 1 edition, February 2010.

[58] G. Klein and D. Murray. Full-3D Edge Tracking with a Particle Filter. In *Proceedings of British Machine Vision Conference*, 2006.

[59] J. Krüger and R. Westermann. Linear algebra operators for GPU implementation of numerical algorithms. In *SIGGRAPH '03: ACM SIGGRAPH 2003 Papers*, pages 908–916, New York, NY, USA, 2003. ACM.

[60] Sheetal Lahabar, Pinky Agarwal, and P.J.Narayanan. High performance pattern recognition on gpu. In *NCVPRIPG: National Conference on Computer Vision, Pattern recognition, Image Processing and Graphics*, Gandhinagar, Gujarat, India, 2008.

[61] P. Lanvin, J.-C. Noyer, and M. Benjelloun. An hardware architecture for 3D object tracking and motion estimation. In *Proceedings of International Conference on Multimedia and Expo (ICME)*, 2005.

[62] E. S. Larsen and D. McAllister. Fast matrix multiplies using graphics hardware. In *Proceedings of the 2001 ACM/IEEE conference on Supercomputing (Supercomputing '01)*, pages 55–55, New York, NY, USA, 2001. ACM.

[63] A. E. Lefohn. A streaming narrow-band algorithm: Interactive computation and visualization of level-set surfaces. Master's thesis, University of Utah, 2003.

[64] A. E. Lefohn, J. E. Cates, and R. T. Whitaker. Interactive, GPU-Based Level Sets for 3D Segmentation. In *Proceedings of the Medical Image Computing and Computer Assisted Intervention (MICCAI)*, 2003.

[65] A.E. Lefohn, J. E. Cates, and R. T. Whitaker. Interactive, GPU-Based Level Sets for 3D Brain Tumor Segmentation. Technical report, School of Computing, University of Utah, 2003.

[66] C. Lenz, G. Panin, and A. Knoll. A GPU-accelerated particle filter with pixel-level likelihood. In *Proceedings of the International Workshop on Vision Modeling and Visualization (VMV '08)*, 2008.

[67] M. Li, M. Magnor, and H. Seidel. Hardware-Accelerated Visual Hull Reconstruction and Rendering. In *Proceedings of Graphics Interface 2003*, pages 65–71, 2003.

[68] P. Li and L. Xiao. Mean Shift Parallel Tracking on GPU. In *Proceedings of the 4th Iberian Conference on Pattern Recognition and Image Analysis (IbPRIA '09)*, pages 120–127, Berlin, Heidelberg, 2009. Springer-Verlag.

[69] W. Li, X. Wei, and A. Kaufman. Implementing Lattice Boltzmann Computation on Graphics Hardware. *The Visual Computer*, 19:444–456, 2003.

[70] O. M. Lozano and K. Otsuka. Real-time Visual Tracker by Stream Processing. *Journal of Signal Processing Systems*, 2008.

[71] Zhongwen Luo, Hongzhi Liu, and Xincai Wu. Artificial neural network computation on graphic process unit. In *IJCNN '05: Proceedings of the 2005 IEEE International Joint Conference on Neural Networks*, pages 622–626, Montreal, Canada, August 2005.

[72] W. Manuel, P. Thomas, U. Markus, and B. Horst. A Variational Model for Interactive Shape Prior Segmentation and Real-Time Tracking. In *Proceedings of the International Conference on Scale Space and Variational Methods in Computer Vision (SSVM 2009)*, 2009.

[73] M. Martínez-Zarzuela, F. Díaz-Pernas, M. Antón-Rodríguez, J. Díez-Higuera, D. González-Ortega, and Boto-Giralda. Multi-scale neural texture classification using the gpu as a stream processing engine. *MMach. Vision Appl.*, March 2010.

[74] M. Martínez-Zarzuela, F. J. Díaz Pernas, J. F. Díez Higuera, and M. Antón-Rodríguez. Fuzzy art neural network parallel computing on the gpu. In Francisco Sandoval Hernández, Alberto Prieto, Joan Cabestany, and Manuel Graña, editors, *IWANN*, volume 4507 of *Lecture Notes in Computer Science*, pages 463–470. Springer, 2007.

[75] M. Martínez-Zarzuela, F.J. Díaz-Pernas, A. Tejero de Pablos, M. Antón-Rodríguez, J. Fernando Díez Higuera, D. Boto-Giralda, and D. González Ortega. Adaptive resonance theory fuzzy networks parallel computation using cuda. In Joan Cabestany, Manuel Graña Francisco Sandoval Hernández, and Alberto Prieto and, editors, *IWANN*, volume 5517 of *Lecture Notes in Computer Science*, pages 150–157. Springer, 2009.

[76] J. L. Mitchell, M. Y. Ansari, and E. Hart. *ShaderX2: Shader Programming Tips and Tricks with DirectX 9.0*, chapter Advanced image processing with DirectX 9 pixel shaders, pages 457–464. Wordware Publishing, 2002.

[77] Y. Mizukami and K. Tadamura. Optical Flow Computation on Compute Unified Device Architecture. In *Proceedings of The 14th International Conference on Image Analysis and Processing (ICIAP '07)*, 2007.

[78] A. S. Montemayor, J. J. Pantrigo, A. Sánchez, and F. Fernández. Particle Filter on GPUs for Real Time Tracking. In *SIGGRAPH '04: ACM SIGGRAPH 2004 posters*, 2004.

[79] A. S. Montemayor, J. J. Pantrigo, A. Sánchez, and F. Fernández. Particle Filter on GPUs for Multiple Object Tracking in HCI Applications. In *SIGGRAPH '05: ACM SIGGRAPH 2005 posters*, 2005.

[80] Á. Moravánszky and A. Novodex. Dense matrix algebra on the GPU. In *Direct3D ShaderX2*, page 2. NovodeX AG, 2003.

[81] K. Moreland and E. Angel. The FFT on a GPU. In *Proceedings of the ACM SIGGRAPH/EUROGRAPHICS conference on Graphics hardware (HWWS '03)*, 2003.

[82] E. Murphy-Chutorian and M. M. Trivedi. Particle filtering with rendered models: A two pass approach to multi-object 3D tracking with the GPU. In *Proceedings of Visual Computer Vision on GPUs (CVGPU '08)*, page 8, 2008.

[83] Jayram Moorkanikara Nageswaran, Nikil Dutt, Jeffrey L Krichmar, Alex Nicolau, and Alex Veidenbaum. Efficient simulation of large-scale spiking neural networks using graphics processors. In *IJCNN*, 2009.

[84] NVIDIA. CUDA Zone. http://www.nvidia.com/object/cuda_home.html, 2008.

[85] NVIDIA. Cuda data-parallel primitives library (CUDPP). `http://gpgpu.org/developer/cudpp`, 2009.

[86] NVIDIA. Nvidia cuda best practices guide 3.0. Technical report, NVIDIA, 2010.

[87] NVIDIA. Nvidia cuda programming guide 3.0. Technical report, NVIDIA, 2010.

[88] *Nvision 2008*, San José, CA, 2008.

[89] K. Oh and Keechul Jung. Gpu implementation of neural networks. *Pattern Recognition*, 37(6):1311–1314, June 2004.

[90] J. D. Owens, D. Luebke, N. Govindaraju, M. Harris, J. Krüger, A. E. Lefohn, and T. J. Purcell. A Survey of General-Purpose Computation on Graphics Hardware. In *Proceedings of Eurographics 2005, State of the Art Reports*, pages 21–51, 2005.

[91] J. D. Owens, S. Sengupta, and D. Horn. Assessment of Graphic Processing Units (GPUs) for Department of Defense (DoD) Digital Signal Processing (DSP) Applications. Technical report, University of California, 2005.

[92] John D. Owens. Streaming architectures and tecnology trends. In Matt Pharr, editor, *GPU Gems 2*, chapter 29, pages 457–470. Addison Wesley, 2005.

[93] John D. Owens, Mike Houston, David Luebke, Simon Green, John E. Stone, and James C. Phillips. GPU computing. *Proceedings of the IEEE*, 96(5):879–899, May 2008.

[94] John D. Owens, David Luebke, Naga Govindaraju, Mark Harris, Jens Krüger, Aaron E. Lefohn, and Timothy J. Purcell. A survey of general-purpose computation on graphics hardware. *Computer Graphics Forum*, 26(1):80–113, 2007.

[95] S. G. Rao and L. F. Hodges. Interactive marker-less tracking of human limbs. Technical report, University of North Carolina Charlotte, 2005.

[96] Thomas Rolfes. Artificial neural networks on programmable graphics hardware. In *Game Programming Gems 4 (Game Programming Gems Series)*. Charles River Media, Inc., Rockland, MA, USA, 2004.

[97] M. Rumpf and R. Strzodka. Level Set Segmentation in Graphics Hardware. In *Proceedings of the IEEE International Conference on Image Processing (ICIP'01)*, 2001.

[98] M. Rumpf and R. Strzodka. Using Graphics Cards for Quantized FEM Computations. In *Proceedings of IASTED Visualization, Imaging and Image Processing Conference (VIIP '01)*, pages 193–202, 2001.

[99] T. Schiwietz and R. Westermann. GPU-PIV. In *Proceedings of Vision, Modeling, and Visualization*, 2004.

[100] Shubhabrata Sengupta, Aaron E. Lefohn, and John D. Owens. A work-efficient step-efficient prefix sum algorithm. In *Proceedings of the 2006 Workshop on Edge Computing Using New Commodity Architectures*, pages D–26–27, May 2006.

[101] A. Sherbondy, M. Houston, and S. Napel. Fast Volume Segmentation With Simultaneous Visualization Using Programmable Graphics Hardware. In *Proceedings of IEEE Visualization*, 2003.

[102] Dave Steinkrau, Patrice Y. Simard, and Ian Buck. Using gpus for machine learning algorithms. In *ICDAR '05: Proceedings of the Eighth International Conference on Document Analysis and Recognition*, pages 1115–1119, Washington, DC, USA, 2005. IEEE Computer Society.

[103] R. Strzodka, M. Droske, and M. Rumpf. Image Registration by a Regularized Gradient Flow - A Streaming Implementation in DX9 Graphics Hardware. *Computing*, 73(4):373–389, November 2004.

[104] R. Strzodka, I. Ihrke, and M. Magnor. A Graphics Hardware Implementation of the Generalized Hough Transform for fast Object Recognition, Scale, and 3D Pose Detection. In *Proceedings of IEEE International Conference on Image Analysis and Processing (ICIAP '03)*, pages 188–193, 2003.

[105] T. Sumanaweera and D. Liu. Medical Image Reconstruction with the FFT. In M. Pharr, editor, *GPU Gems 2: Programming Techniques for High-Performance Graphics and General-Purpose Computation*. Addison-Wesley Publishing Company, 2005.

[106] P. Thomas, G. Markus, and B. Horst. Real-time Computation of Variational Methods on Graphics Hardware. In *Proceedings of the Computer Vision Winter Workshop*, 2007.

[107] C. J. Thompson, S. Hahn, and M. Oskin. Using Modern Graphics Architectures for General-Purpose Computing: A Framework and Analysis. In *Proceedings of the International Symposium on Microarchitecture (MICRO)*, 2002.

[108] V. Vineet and P. J. Narayanan. CUDA Cuts: Fast Graph Cuts on the GPU In. In *Proceedings of IEEE Computer Society Conference on Computer Vision and Pattern Recognition Workshops*, 2008.

[109] John Von Neumann. First draft of a report on the edvac. Technical report, 1945.

[110] M. M. Wloka. Implementing a GPU-Efficient FFT. In D. Manocha, editor, *ACM SIGGRAPH "Interactive Geometric & Scientific Computations with Graphics Hardware" Course Notes*, pages 132–137, 2003.

[111] R. Yang and M. Pollefeys. Multi-Resolution Real-Time Stereo on Commodity Graphics Hardware. In *Proceedings of the IEEE Computer Society Conference on Computer Vision and Pattern Recognition (CVPR '03)*, 2003.

[112] R. Yang and G. Welch. Fast Image Segmentation and Smoothing Using Commodity Graphics Hardware. *Journal of Graphics Tools*, 7(4):91–100, 2002.

[113] R. Yang, G. Welch, and G. Bishop. Real-Time Consensus-Based Scene Reconstruction using Commodity Graphics Hardware, 2002.

[114] C. Zeller. Cloth simulation on the GPU. In *SIGGRAPH '05: ACM SIGGRAPH 2005 Sketches*, page 39, New York, NY, USA, 2005. ACM.

In: Computer Graphics
Editor: Martin J. Davis
ISBN: 978-1-61761-811-6

Chapter 8

FRACTAL GEOMETRY IN COMPUTER GRAPHICS AND IN VIRTUAL REALITY*

Nicoletta Sala†
[1]Accademia di Architettura, Università della Svizzera Italiana, Largo Bernasconi, Mendrisio, Switzerland
[2]Dipartimento di Informatica e Comunicazione Università dell'Insubria, Via Mazzini 5, Varese, Italy

ABSTRACT

Fractal geometry is also known as "Mandelbrot's geometry" in honour to its "father" the mathematician Benoit Mandelbrot (b. 1924), that showed how fractals can occur in many different places in mathematics and in other disciplines. Fractal geometry can be used for modelling natural shapes (e.g., fern, trees, seashells, rivers, mountains), and its important applications also appear in computer science, because this "new" geometry permits to compress the images, to reproduce, in the virtual reality environments, the complex patterns and the irregular forms present in nature using simple iterative instructions. The aim of this paper is to present the applications of fractal geometry in computer graphics (to compress images) and in virtual reality (to generate virtual territories and landscapes).

Keywords: Fractal Geometry, Self-Similarity, Iterated Function Systems, L-Systems, Fractional Brownian Motion, Computer Graphics, Virtual Reality, Virtual World.

---

* A version of this chapter was also published in *Progress in Chaos and Complexity Research,* edited by Franco F. Orsucci, and Nicoletta Sala, published by Nova Science Publishers, Inc. It was submitted for appropriate modifications in an effort to encourage wider dissemination of research.

† E-mail: nsala@arch.unisi.ch.

1. Introduction

French mathematicians Pierre Fatou (1878-1929) and Gaston Julia (1893-1978) worked on fractals at the beginning of the 20th century. The word "Fractal" was coined by the Polish-born Franco-American Benoit Mandelbrot, and it derives from the Latin verb "frangere", "to break", and from the related adjective "fractus", "fragmented and irregular". This term denotes the geometry of nature, which traces inherent order in chaotic shapes and processes, and it was created to differentiate pure geometric figures from other types of figures that defy such simple classification. The Encyclopaedia Britannica introduces the fractal geometry as follow (2007): "In mathematics, the study of complex shapes with the property of self-similarity, known as fractals. Rather like holograms that store the entire image in each part of the image, any part of a fractal can be repeatedly magnified, with each magnification resembling all or part of the original fractal. This phenomenon can be seen in objects like snowflakes and tree bark… This new system of geometry has had a significant impact on such diverse fields as physical chemistry, physiology, and fluid mechanics; fractals can describe irregularly shaped objects or spatially nonuniform phenomena that cannot be described by Euclidean geometry".

The acceptance of the word "fractal" was dated in 1975, when Mandelbrot presented the list of publications between 1951 and 1975, date when the French version of his book was published, the people were surprised by the variety of the studied fields: economy, linguistics, cosmology, noise on telephone lines, turbulence (Mandelbrot, 1975).

Mandelbrot's geometry replaces Euclidian geometry (which dominated our mathematical thinking for thousands of years) and it is recognized as the true geometry able to describe the Nature. Recently, the electronics evolution and the increase in the computer calculation power permitted connections between the fractal geometry and the other disciplines (for example, biology, economy, medicine, engineering, arts, architecture), and the multiplicity of applications had an important role in the diffusion of fractal geometry (Mandelbrot, 1982; Leland et al., 1993; Nonnenmacker et al., 1994; Eglash, 1999; Barnsley et al., 2002; Sala, 2006; Vyzantiadou et al., 2007). This paper is organized as follows: section 2 introduces the fractal objects, section 3 presents the application of the fractal geometry in computer graphics. Section 4 introduces the fractal geometry as a tool for modelling virtual landscapes. Section 5 is dedicated to the conclusions.

2. Fractal Objects

A fractal object could be defined as a fragmented geometric shape that can be subdivided in parts, each of which is approximately a reduced-size copy of the whole (Mandelbrot, 1982). Fractals are generally self-similar on multiple scales. So, all fractals have a built-in form of iteration or recursion. Sometimes the recursion is visible in how the fractal is constructed. For example, Koch snowflake, Cantor set, and the Sierpinski triangle (figure 1a) are all generated using simple recursive rules. Self similarity is present in nature, too. Figures 1b shows a natural fractal object, the cauliflower which has the property of self similarity (it repeats its shape in different scales).

The self similarity and other kinds of fractals (e.g., Iterated Function Systems and the Lindenmayer System) are applied in different fields of computer science, for example, in computer graphics, in virtual reality, and in the computer networks (for controlling the traffic) (Leland et al, 1992; Erramilli et al., 1993; Liu, 2006).

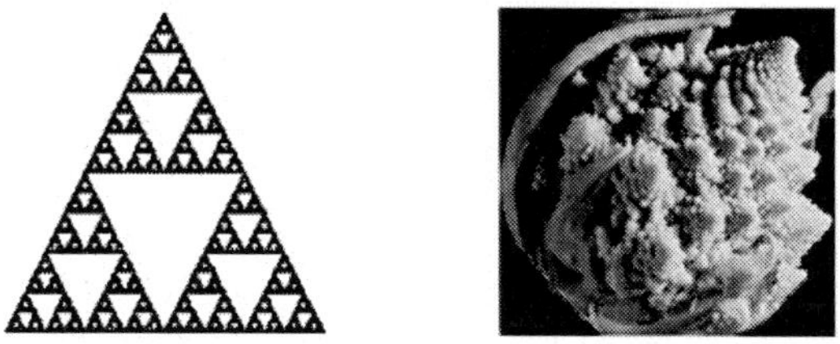

a) b)

Figure 1. The Sierpinski triangle is a fractal generated using simple geometric rules a). The cauliflower is a fractal present in the nature b).

2.1. The Self-Similarity

The invariance against changes in scale or size is named "self-similarity", and it is a property by which an object contains smaller copies of itself at arbitrary scales. Mandelbrot defined the self-similarity as follow: "When each piece of a shape is geometrically similar to the whole, both the shape and the cascade that generate it are called self-similar" (Mandelbrot, 1982, p. 34). "Similar" means that the relative proportions of the internal angles and shapes' sides remain the same. Mandelbrot (1982) observed that this property is ubiquitous in the natural world, and in the human body is possible to observe the presence of fractal geometry using two different points of view: temporal fractals and spatial fractals.

Temporal fractals are present in some dynamic processes, for example in the cardiac rhythm. Spatial fractals refer to the presence of self-similarity observed to various enlargements, for instance, the small intestine repeats its form on different scales. Spatial fractals also refer to the branched patterns that are present inside the human body for enlarging the available surface for the absorption of the substances, and the distribution and the collection of the solutes occupying a relative small fraction of the body.

Figure 2a above shows the frontal view of dog's lungs. It is an example of self-similarity in the nature. In figures 2b there is an example of a fractal object which represents an attempt to reproduce complex shapes of the lungs, using few simple geometric rules.

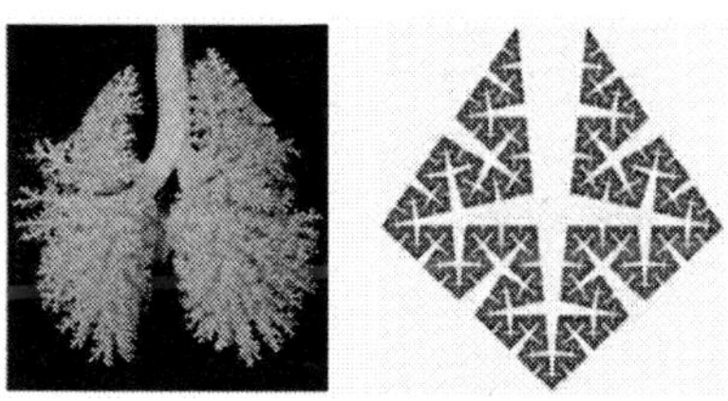

a) b)

Figure 2. Frontal view of dog's lungs a) it is a natural fractal object. "Fractal lungs" b) is a fractal generated using simple geometric rules, starting from two triangles.

2.2. The Iterated Function System

Iterated Function System (IFS) is another fractal that can be applied in computer science, in particular in computer graphics. Barnsley (1993, p. 80) defined the Iterated Function System as follow: "A (hyperbolic) iterated function system consists of a complete metric space (X, d) together with a finite set of contraction mappings w_n: X→ X with respective contractivity factor s_n, for n = 1, 2,.., N. The abbreviation "IFS" is used for "iterated function system". The notation for the IFS just announced is {X, w_n, n = 1, 2,.., N} and its contractivity factor is $s = \max\{s_n : n = 1, 2, \ldots, N\}$." Barnsley put the word "hyperbolic" in parentheses because it is sometimes dropped in practice. He also defined the following theorem (Barnsley, 1993, p. 81): "Let {X, w_n, n = 1, 2, …, N} be a hyperbolic iterated function system with contractivity factor s. Then the transformation W: H(**X**) → H(**X**) defined by:

$$W(B) = \cup_{n=1}^{n} w_n(B) \quad (1)$$

For all B∈ H(X), is a contraction mapping on the complete metric space (H(X), h(d)) with contractivity factor s. That is:

$$H(W(B), W(C)) \leq s \cdot h(B,C) \quad (2)$$

$$A = W(A) = \cup_{n=1}^{n} w_n(A) \quad (3)$$

for all B, C ∈ H(**X**). Its unique fixed point, A ∈ H(X), obeys and is given by $A = \lim_{n\to\infty} W^{on}(B)$ for any B ∈ H(X)."

The fixed point A ∈ H(X), described in the theorem by Barnsley is called the "attractor of the IFS" or "invariant set".

An affine map of the plane is given by form:

$$w\begin{bmatrix} x \\ y \end{bmatrix} = \begin{bmatrix} a & c \\ b & d \end{bmatrix}\begin{bmatrix} x \\ y \end{bmatrix} + \begin{bmatrix} e \\ f \end{bmatrix}$$

and it is determined by six number, a, b, c, d, e, and f. The affine maps are combinations of translations, rotations and scalings in the plane. If the scaling factor is less than 1, we have contractive affine maps.

Bogomolny (1998) affirms that two problems arise. One is to determine the fixed point of a given IFS, and it is solved by what is known as the "*deterministic* algorithm".

The second problem is the inverse of the first: for a given set A∈H(X), find an iterated function system that has A as its fixed point (Bogomolny, 1998). This is solved approximately by the Collage Theorem (Barnsley, 1993, p. 94).

The Collage Theorem states: “Let (X, d), be a complete metric space. Let L∈H(X) be given, and let $\varepsilon \geq o$ be given. Choose an IFS (or IFS with condensation) $\{X, (w_n), w_1, w_2, \ldots, w_n\}$ with contractivity factor $0 \leq s \leq 1$, so that

$$h(L, \cup_{n=1 \atop (n=0)}^{n} w_n(L)) \leq \varepsilon \qquad (4)$$

where h(d) is the Hausdorff metric. Then

$$h(L, A) \leq \frac{\varepsilon}{1-s} \qquad (5)$$

where A is the attractor of the IFS. Equivalently

$$h(L, A) \leq (1-s)^{-1} h(L, \cup_{n-1 \atop (n-0)} w_n(L)) \qquad (6)$$

for all L∈H(X).”

The Collage Theorem describes how to find an Iterated Function System whose attractor is “close to” a given set, one must endeavour to find a set of transformations such that the union, or collage, of the images of the given set under transformations is near to the given set.

2.3. L-Systems

Hungarian biologist Aristid Lindenmayer (1925-1989) introduced a kind of fractals, called L-systems, for modelling biological growth in 1968. L-system or Lindenmayer system is an algorithmic method for generating branched forms and structures such as plants. The components of an L-system are the following:

- An alphabet which is a finite set V of formal symbols containing elements that can be replaced (variables).
- the constants which is a set S of symbols containing elements that remain fixed.
- The *axiom* (also called the *initiator*) which is a string ω of symbols from V defining the initial state of the system.
- A *production* (or *rewriting rule*) P that is a set of rules or productions defining the way variables can be replaced with combinations of constants and other variables. A production consists of two strings - the predecessor and the successor.

The rules of the L-system grammar are applied iteratively starting from the initial state.

L-systems are also commonly known as parametric L systems, and they are defined as a tuple $G = \{V, S, \omega, P\}$. L-system can be also defined as a formal grammar (a set of rules and symbols) most famously used for modelling the growth processes of plant development, and it has been thought able for modelling the morphology of a variety of organisms. The differences between L-systems and Chomsky grammars are well described by Prusinkiewicz and Lindenmayer that affirmed: "The essential difference between Chomsky grammars and L-systems lies in the method of applying productions. In Chomsky grammars productions are applied sequentially, whereas in L-systems they are applied in parallel and simultaneously replace all letters in a given word. This difference highlights the biological motivation of L-systems. Productions are intended to capture cell divisions in multicellular organisms, where many divisions may occur at the same time. Parallel production application has an essential impact on the formal properties of rewriting systems" (Prusinkiewicz and Lindenmayer, 1990, pp. 2 – 3). Strings generated by L-systems may be interpreted geometrically in different ways.

Table 1. Commands for LOGO-style turtle derived by L-systems

Symbols	Meaning
F	Move forward a step of length s. The state of the turtle changes, now it is (x', y', α), where x' = x +s ·cos α and y'= y + s ·sin α. A segment between (x, y), starting point, and the point (x', y') is drawn.
f	Move forward a tep of length s without drawing a line.
+	Turn left by angle δ. The positive orientation of angles is counterclockwise, and the next state of the turtle is (x, y, $\alpha+\delta$).
-	Turn right by angle δ. The next state of the turtle is (x, y, α - δ).
[	Push the current state of the turtle onto a pushdown operations stack. The information saved on the stack contains the turtle's position and orientation, and possibly other attributes such as the color and width of lines being drawn.
]	Pop a state from the stack and make it the current state of the turtle. No line is drawn, although in general the position of the turtle changes.

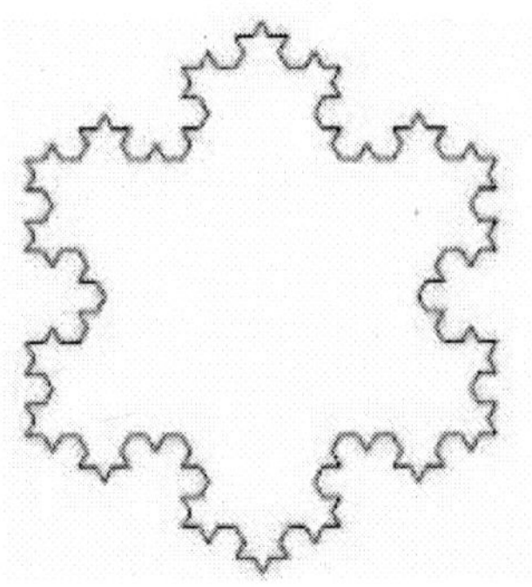

Figure 3. Koch snowflake generated by L-system.

For example, L-system strings serve a drawing commands for LOGO-style turtle. Prusinkiewicz and Lindenmayer defined a state of the turtle as a triplet (x, y, α), where the Cartesian coordinates (x, y) represent the turtle's position, and the angle α, called the heading, is interpreted as the direction in which the turtle is facing. Given the step size s and the angle increment δ, the turtle can respond to commands represented by the symbols in the table 1 above.

The Koch snowflake can be simply encoded as a Lindenmayer system with initial string "F++F++F", string rewriting rule F → F-F++F-F, and angle 60°, as shown in figure 3.

3. Fractal Geometry in Computer Graphics

The terms fractals has been generalized by the computer graphics community and it includes objects outside Mandelbrot's original definition (Foley et al., 1997). It means anything that has a substantial measure of exact or statistical self-similarity. In the case of statistical fractals it is the probability density that repeats itself on every scale. An application field of fractal geometry is in the compression of images (fractal compression). A fractal compressed image can be defined as follow: it is an encoding that describes (i) the grid partitioning (the range blocks), and (ii) the affine transformations (one per range block) (Shulman, 2000). Research on fractal image compression derived from the mathematical ferment on chaos and fractals in the years 1978–1985. Barnsley was the principal researcher who worked in this field. The basic idea was to represent by an Iterated Function System (IFS) of which the fixed point is close to that image (Barnsley, 1988; Barnsley et al., 1988). This fixed point is also known as "fractal" (Fisher, 1995). Each IFS is coded as a contractive transformation with coefficients. The Banach fixed point theorem (1922), also known as the contraction mapping theorem or contraction mapping principle, guarantees the existence and uniqueness of fixed points of certain self maps of metric spaces, and provides a constructive method to find those fixed points.

An image can be represented using a set of IFS codes rather than pixels. In this way, a good compression ratio could be achieved. This method was good for generating almost real images based on simple iterative algorithms. The inverse problem, going from a given image to an Iterated Function System that can generate the original (or at least closely resemble it), was solved by Jacquin according to Barnsley in March 1988. He introduced a modified scheme for representing images called Partitioned Iterated Function Systems (PIFS). The main characteristics of this approach were that (i) it relied on the assumption that image redundancy can be efficiently exploited through self-transformability on a block-wise basis, and (ii) it approximated an original image by a fractal image (Jacquin, 1992). In a PIFS, the transformations do not map from the whole image to the parts, but from larger parts to smaller parts. In the Jacquin's method, the small areas are called "range blocks", the big areas are called "domain blocks" and the pattern of range blocks was called the "partitioning of an image". Every pixel of the original image has to belong to one range block. This system of mappings is contractive, thus when iterated it quickly converge to its fixed point image. Thus, the key point for this algorithm is to find fractals which can best describe the original image and then to represent them as affine transformations.

All methods are based on the fractal transform using iterated function systems which generate a close approximation of a scene using only few transformations (Peitgen and Saupe, 1988; Wohlberg and de Jager, 1999; Zhao and Liu, 2005).

Fractal compression is a lossy compression method (compressing data and then decompressing it retrieves data that may well be different from the original, but is close enough to be useful in some way), and most lossy compression formats suffer from generation loss: repeatedly compressing and decompressing the file will cause it to progressively lose quality (as shown in figure 4).

In the field of the compression of images novel methods are studied. For example, van Wijk and Saupe (2004) present a fast method to generate fractal imagery based on Iterated Function Systems. The high performance derives from three factors: (i) all steps are expressed in graphics operations which can be performed quickly by hardware, (ii) frame to frame coherence is exploited, (iii) only a few commands per image have to be passed from the CPU to the graphics hardware, avoiding the classical CPU bottleneck.

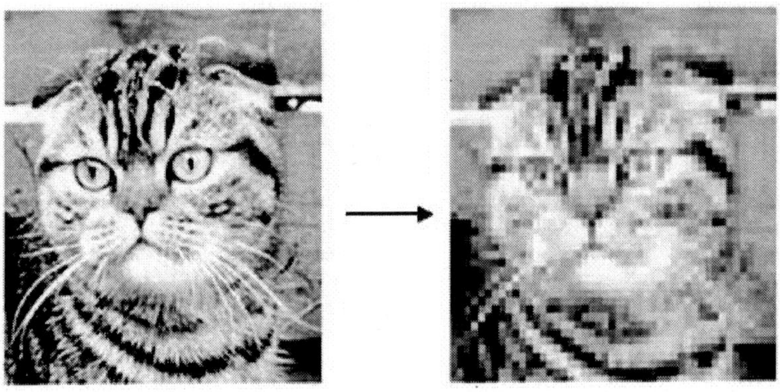

Figure 4. Fractal compression: repeatedly compressing and decompressing the file will cause it to progressively lose quality.

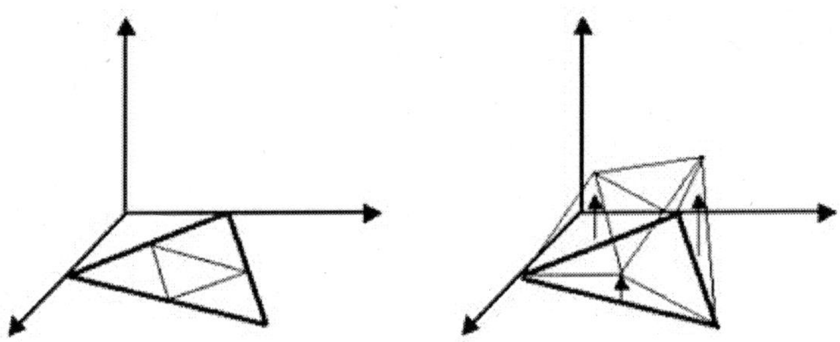

a) b)

Figure 5. The subdivision of a triangle into four smaller triangle a). Perturbation in the y direction of the midpoints of the original triangle b).

4. Fractal Geometry for Modelling Virtual Landscapes

Other interesting application of fractal geometry in computer science is for modelling landscapes which include terrain, mountains, trees and so forth. Fournier et al. *(1982) developed a mechanism for generating a kind of fractal mountains based on recursive subdivision* algorithm for a triangle. Here, the midpoints of each side of the triangle are connected, creating four new subtriangles. Figure 5a shows the subdivision of the triangle into four smaller triangle, figure 5b illustrates how the midpoints of the original triangle are perturbed in the y direction (Foley et al., 1997). To perturb these points, can be use the properties of the self-similarity, and the conditional expectation properties of fractional Brownian motion (abbreviated to fBm). The fractional Brownian motion was originally introduced by Mandelbrot and Van Ness in 1968 as a generalization of the Brownian motion (Bm). FBm basically consists of steps in a random direction and with a step-length that has some characteristic value. Hence the random walk process. An important feature of fBm is the self-similarity (if we zoom in on any part of the function we will produce a similar random walk in the zoomed in part). Figure 6 shows a recursive subdivision of an initial polygon using squares. Other polygons can be used to generate the grid (e.g., triangles and hexagons).

This method evidences two problems, which are classified as internal and external consistency problems (Fournier et al., 1982, pp. 374-375). Internal consistency is the reproducibility of the primitive at any position in an appropriate coordinate space and at any level of detail, so the final shape is independent of the orientation of the subdivided triangle. This is satisfied by a Gaussian random number generator which depends on the point's position, thus it generates the same numbers in the same order at a given subdivision level. The external consistency concerns the midpoint displacement at shared edges and their direction of displacement. This process, when iterated, produces a deformed grid which represents a surface, an example is shown in figure 6. After the rendering phase (that includes: hidden line, coloured, and shaded) can appear a realistic fractal mountain, as shown in figure 7.

Their method created one non-branching river as result of context sensitive L-system operating on geometric objects (a set of triangles). Three key problems remained open (i) the river flowed at a constant altitude, (ii) the river flowed in an asymmetric valley, and (iii) the river had no tributaries. Figure 8 shows an example of a squig-curve construction (recursion levels 0–7) (Prusinkiewicz and Hammel, 1993, p. 177).

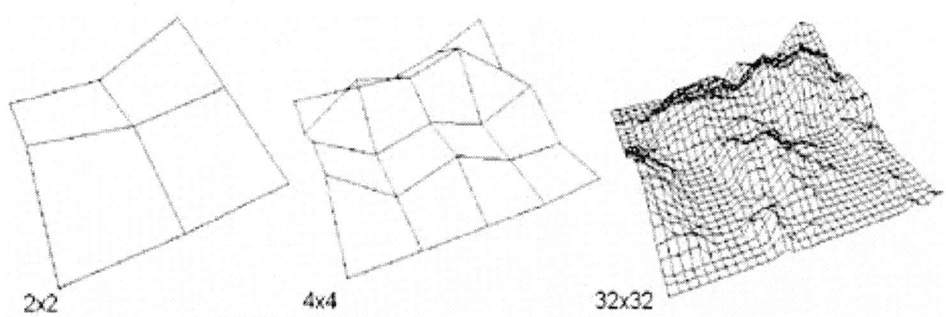

Figure 6. Grid of squares generated by a recursive subdivision and applying the fractional Brownian motion.

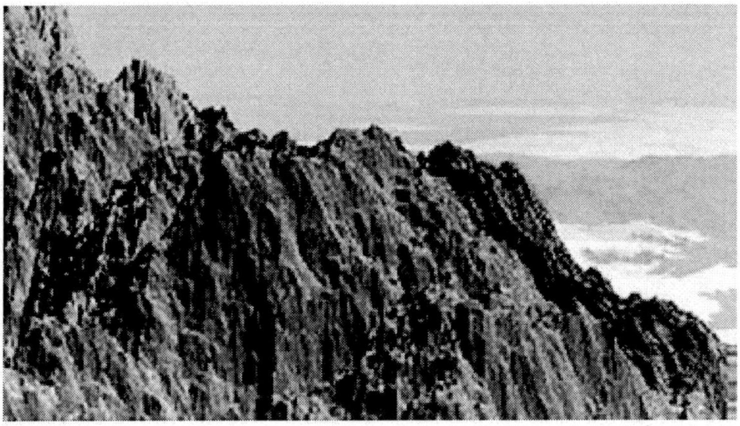

Figure 7. Fractal mountains.

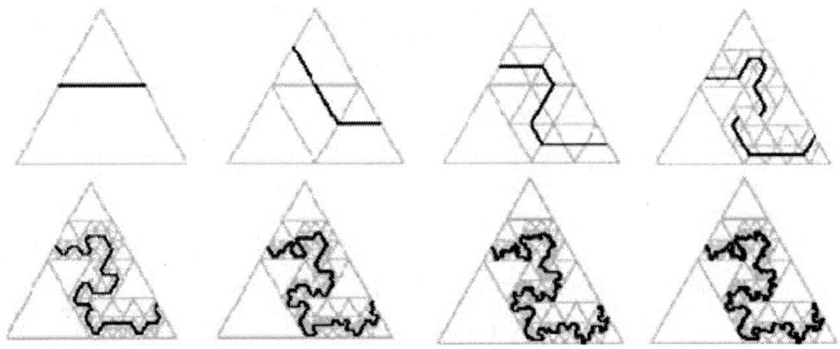

Figure 8. Squid-curve construction (recursion level 0-7).

Maràk et al. (1997) reported a method for synthetical terrain erosion, that is based on rewriting process of matrices representing terrain parts. They found a rewriting process which was context sensitive. It was defined as a set of productions $A \rightarrow B$, where A and B were matrices of numbers of type: $N \times N$, where $N>0$.

The terrain parts were rewritten using certain user-defined set of rules which represented an erosion process. The method consisted in three kinds of rewriting process (Maràk et al., 1997; Maràk, 1997). The "absolute rewriting" which permitted to erode the objects in predefined altitude.

The "rewriting with the reference point" which could erode arbitrary object in any altitude. The third kind of rewriting process which permitted to erode some shapes in any scale. Its advantage was that the algorithm could be controlled by some external rules and it could simulate different kinds of erosion (Maràk et al., 1997).

Fractal algorithms can also be used in computer graphics to generate complex objects using Iterated Function Systems. Figure 9 shows a fern leaf created using the IFS. The IFS is produced by polygons, in this case: squares, that are put in one another. The final step of this iterative process shows a fern which has high degree of similarity to real one.

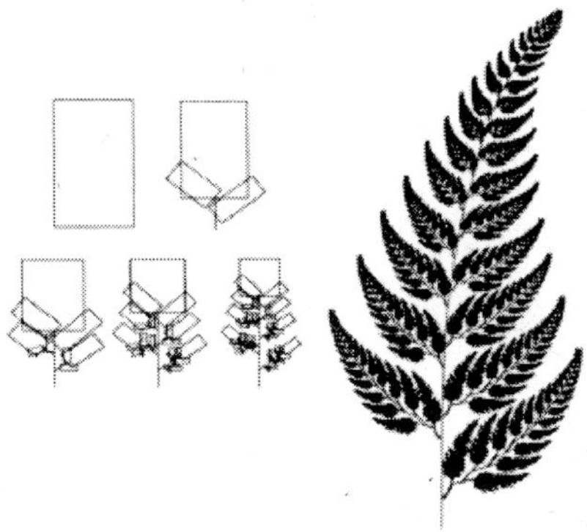

Figure 9. Fern leaf created using the IFS.

Originally the L-systems were devised to provide a formal description of the development of such simple multicellular organisms, and to illustrate the neighbourhood relationships between plant cells. Later on, this system was extended to describe higher plants and complex branching structures. Smith (1984) was the first to prove that L-systems were useful in computer graphics for describing the structure of certain plants, in his paper: "Plants, Fractals, and Formal Languages". He described that these objects should not be labeled as "fractals" for their similarity to fractals, introducing a new class of objects which Smith called "graftals".

This class had of great interest in the Computer Imagery (Smith, 1984; Foley et al., 1997). Figure 10 shows an example of plant-like structures generated after four iterations by bracketed L-systems with the initial string F (angle $\delta = 22.5°$), and the replacement rule F →FF+[+F-F-F] -[-F+F+F].

Using fractal algorithms is possible to create virtual mountains and virtual trees described in Virtual Reality Modelling Language (VRML), as shown in figure 11a. VRML is a 3D graphics language used on the World Wide Web for producing "virtual worlds" that appear on the display screens using an appropriate VRML browser. This example shows that the connections between fractal geometry, and the "virtual worlds" exit. A virtual world is a computer-based simulated environment intended for its users to inhabit and interact via avatars. Avatars can walk on virtual territory generated with fractal algorithms. Figure 11b shows a fractal tree generated with simple geometric iterative rules.

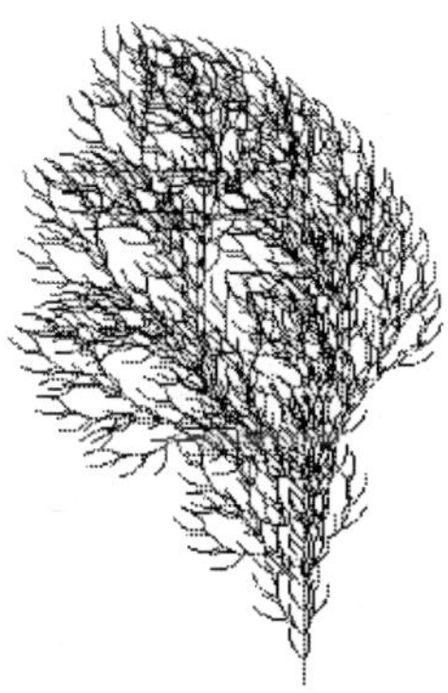

Figure 10. Plant-like structures generated after four iterations by bracketed L-systems.

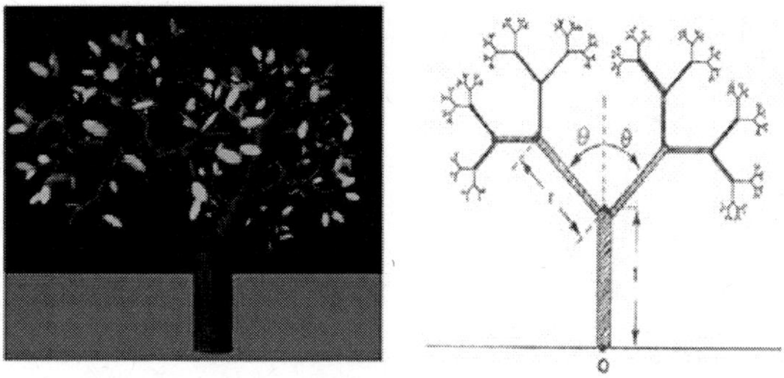

a) b)

Figure 11. Virtual tree realized in VRML using fractal algorithms a). A fractl geometric tree b).

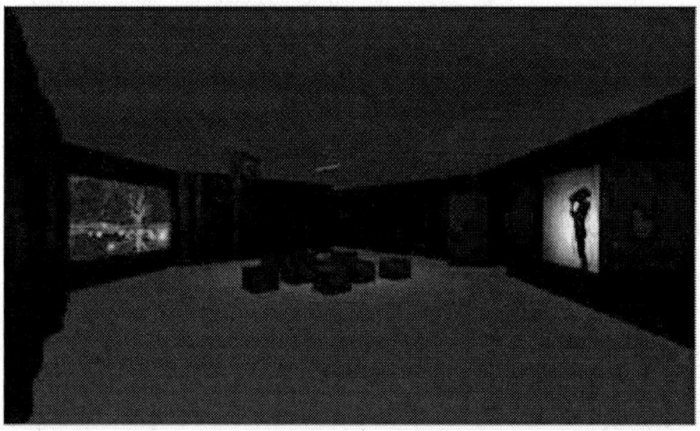

Figure 12. The installation space for *Osmose (1995)*. Char Davies/Immersence Inc.and Softimage Inc.©.

The evolution of the computer graphics techniques and virtual reality technologies, also connected to the fractal algorithms, help to create a new kind of digital arts. Some artists represent a broad range of approaches to installation and virtual reality art (Wands, 2006). For example, Char Davies is a pioneer of this art form. She describes her immersive virtual reality environments *Osmose* (1995) and *Ephémère* (1998) as works "known for their embodying interface, painterly aesthetic and evocation of landscape".

Figure 12 shows the installation space for Osmose. Davies and Harrison claim: "*Osmose* is an immersive virtual environment, produced by Softimage in 1994/95. One of the primary goals of *Osmose* was to push the expressive capabilities of existing 3D tools, to demonstrate that an alternative aesthetic and interactive sensibility is possible for real-time, interactive, 3D computer graphics. *Osmose* was created under the direction of Char Davies, the Director of Visual Research at Softimage.(…) One of Davies' intentions for Osmose was to create a space that is "psychically innovating," one in which, to quote Bachelard, participants do not change "place," but change their own nature. Osmose was therefore designed to explore the potential of immersive virtual space to allow participants to shed their habitual ways of looking at (and behaving in) the world." (Davies and Harrison, p. 25, 1996).

CONCLUSIONS

This paper has described some applications of fractal geometry in computer graphics. The self-similarity, important characteristic of the fractal objects, is a unifying concept, and it is an attribute of many laws of nature and innumerable phenomena in the world around us.

In computer graphics, fractals can be applied in different fields: to compress the images using simple algorithms based on Iterated Function Systems, for modelling complex objects in computer graphics (e.g., mountains, trees and rivers) using L-systems and the fractional Brownian motion. Future trends are oriented to use IFS to generate terrain from real data extracted from geological data base. This is useful in the reconstruction of real terrain and landscapes (Guérin et al., 2002; Guérin, and Tosan, 2005). Fractal geometry also offers an alternative approach to conventional planetary terrain analysis. For example, Stepinski et al. (2004) describe Martian terrains, represented by topography based on the Mars Orbiter Laser Altimetry (MOLA) data, as a series of drainage basins. Fractal analysis of each drainage network, computationally extracts some network descriptors that are used for a quantitative characterization and classification of Martian surfaces.

The Computer graphics connected to the fractal geometry and to the virtual reality have also given to the digital artists powerful tools and new sources of creative expression (davies and Harrison, 1996; Thwaites, 2005; Wands, 2006).

REFERENCES

Barnsley, M. F. (1988). *Fractals everywhere*. Boston: Academic Press.

Barnsley, M. F. (1993). *Fractals everywhere*. Boston: Academic Press, 2nd edition.

M. F., Barnsley, D. Saupe, & E. R. Vrscay, (Eds.) (2002). *Fractals in Multimedia*. Berlin, Germany: Springer.

Barnsley, M. F., Jacquin, A. E., Malassenet, F., Reuter, L. & Sloane, A. D. (1988). Harnessing chaos for image synthesis. *Siggraph*, 131-140.

Bogomolny, A.(1998). *The Collage Theorem*. Retrieved September 1, 2006, from: http://www.cut-the-knot.org/ctk/ifs.shtml.

Davies, C. & Harrison, J. (1996). Osmose: Towards Broadening the Aesthetics of Virtual Reality. *Computer Graphics (ACM SIGGRAPH)*, Vol. XXX (4) 25-28.

Eglash, R. (1999). *African Fractals: Modern Computing and Indigenous Design*. Piscataway, NJ: Rutgers University Press.

Erramilli, A., Gosby, D. & Willinger, W. (1993). Engineering for Realistic Traffic: A Fractal Analysis of Burstiness. *Proceedings of ITC Special Congress*, Bangalore, India, 1993.

Fisher, Y. (1995). *Fractal Image Compression: Theory and Application*. New York: Springer-Verlag.

Foley, J. D., van Dam, A., Feiner, S. K. & Hughes, J. F. (1997). *Computer Graphics: Principles and Practice. Second Edition in C*. New York: Addison Wesley.

Fournier, A., Fussel, D. & Carpenter, L. (1982). Computer Rendering of Stochastic Models. *Communications of the ACM*, 25, 371-384.

Fractal geometry. (2007). In *Encyclopædia Britannica*. Retrieved February 2, 2007, from Britannica Concise Encyclopedia: http:// concise. britannica. com/ebc/article-93647

97/fractal-geometry.

Guérin, E. & Tosan, E. (2005). Fractal Inverse Problem: Approximation Formulation and Differential Methods. J., Lévy-Véhel, & E. Lutton, (Eds.*). Fractal in Engineering: new trends in theory and applications* (271-285). London: Springer.

Guérin, E., Tosan, E. & Baskurt, A. (2002). Modeling and Approximation of Fractal Surfaces with Projected IFS Attractors". M. M. Novak, (Ed.). *Emergent Nature: Patterns, Growth and Scaling in the Science* (293-303). New Jersey: World Scientific.

Leland,W. E., Taqqu, M. S., Willinger, W. & Wilson, D. V. (1993). On the Self-Similar Nature of Ethernet Traffic. *Proceedings of the ACM/SIGCOMM'93*, (183-193) San Francisco, CA.

Mandelbrot, B. (1975). *Les Objects Fractals. Forme, Hasard et Dimension*, Paris, France : Nouvelle Bibliothèque Scientifique Flammaron.

Mandelbrot, B. (1982). *The Fractal Geometry of Nature*. W.H. Freeman and Company.

Maràk I. (1997). *On Synthetic Terrain Erosion Modeling*: A Survey. Retrieved March 14, 2007, from. http://www.cescg.org/CESCG97/marak/

Marák, I., Benes, B. & Slavík, P. (1997). Terrain Erosion Model Based on Rewriting of Matrices. *Proceedings of WSCG-97*, vol. 2., (341-351).

Musgrave, F. K., Kolb, C. E. & Mace, R. S. (1989). The synthesis and rendering of eroded fractal terrain. *Proceedings of SIGGRAPH '89*, in *Computer Graphics* 23, 3, (pp.41–50), ACM SIGGRAPH, New York.

T. F., Nonnenmacher, G. A., Losa, D. Merlini, & E. R. Weibel, (Eds.). (1994). *Fractal in Biology and Medicine*. Basel, Switzerland: Birkhauser.

Peitgen, H. and Saupe, D. (1988). *The Science of Fractal Images*. New York: Springer-Verlag.

Prusinkiewicz, P. & Hammel, M. (1993). A Fractal Model of Mountains with Rivers. *Proceeding of Graphics Interface '93*, 174-180.

Prusinkiewicz, P. & Lindenmayer, A. (1990). *The Algorithmic Beauty of Plants*. New York, US: Springer-Verlag. Retrieved September 10, 2007, from:
http://algorithmicbotany.org/papers/abop/abop.pdf

Sala, N. (2006). Complexity, Fractals, Nature and Industrial Design: Some Connections, M. M. Novak, (Ed.). *Complexus Mundi: Emergent Pattern in Nature*. (171-180). Singapore: World Scientific.

Stepinski, T. F., Collier, M. L., McGovern, P. J. & Clifford, S. M. (2004). Martian geomorphology from fractal analysis of drainage networks. *Journal of Geophysical Research*, *Vol. 109,* n°E2, E02005.1-E02005.12.

Thwaites, H. (2005). *The Immersant Experience of Osmose and Ephémère."* [PDF File] Proceedings of the 2005 international conference on Augmented tele-existence ICAT '05. Christchurch, New Zealand, 148-155.

van Wijk, J. J. & Saupe D. (2004). Image based rendering of iterated function systems. *Computers and Graphics*, *28(6)*, 937-943.

Vyzantiadou, M. A., Avdelas, A. V. & Zafiropoulos, S. (2007). The application of fractal geometry to the design of grid or reticulated shell structures. *Computer-Aided Design*, *Volume 39*, issue 1, 51-59.

Wands, B. (2006). *Art of the Digital Age*. New York, NY: Thames and Hudson Inc.

Wohlberg, B. & de Jager, G. (1999). A Review of the Fractal Image Coding Literature. *IEEE Transactions on Image Processing*, *8(12)*, 1716-1729.

Zhao, E. & Liu, D. (2005). Fractal image compression methods: a review. ICITA 2005. *Third International Conference on Information Technology and Applications*, *Volume 1* (756-759).

In: Computer Graphics
Editor: Martin J. Davis

ISBN: 978-1-61761-811-6

Chapter 9

VISUAL ATTENTION IN COMPUTER GRAPHICS*

A. Artusi and A. Chalmers*
Warwick Digital Laboratory, University of Warwick, UK

1 Introduction

Visual attention, as part of the visual perception, is the ability of the Human Visual System (HVS) to find and focus on relevant information quickly and efficiently [Re02]. The most important aspect of the visual attention is its capacity to rapidly select objects of interest in our visual environment. Objects which are not perceptually important can often go completely unnoticed [16]. In the HVS, the eyes do not scan a scene in a raster-like fashion, but rather they jump so that important parts of the scene fall sequentially onto the fovea, the area of highest visual acuity within our eyes. There are two distinct visual attention processes, which [19] termed bottom-up and top-down. The bottom-up process is purely stimulus driven. This is evolutionary, enabling our eyes to rapidly identify salient information in a scene without volitional control such as a candle burning in a dark room, saturated colours etc.

The top-down process is, on the other hand, under voluntary control and enables our visual system to focus on parts of a scene which may be relevant to accomplish a task within that scene. Inattentional blindness is a feature of the HVS which may result in objects in a scene which would normally attract attention, being completely ignored if they are not relevant to the current task [16] [24].

Recently human visual attention has been increasingly exploited in computer graphics in order to reduce the significant cost of computing high-fidelity images. By only computing in high quality those areas of a scene which are perceptually important, significant computation time can be saved without the user being aware of the quality differences within the image.

In computer graphics, early work, including the Visual Difference Predictor [7] [17] and the Visible Discrimination Model [3], used knowledge of the HVS to investigate the

*A version of this chapter was also published in Visual Perception: New Research edited by Isak L. Nilsson and William V. Lindberg published by Nova Science Publishers. It was submitted for appropriate modifications in an effort to encourage wider dissemination of research.

perceptual quality of images. Visual attention models have also been used to significantly reduce the overall computation time for global illumination calculations without a perceptible loss of image quality [31] [6]. More recently, researchers have used detailed models of the bottom-up (known as Saliency Maps [12]) and top-down (known as Task Maps [6]) visual attention processes to significantly speed-up the computation of high-fidelity images. More recent work has discovered that the information contained in the traditional Saliency and/or

Tasks maps is often redundant. In particular, this redundant information may not be used in order to accelerate the computation process. However, an extra computation time to compute this redundant information is added on the computation of high-fidelity images either precluding or drastically reducing any speed-up. It is clear that trough undertsanding of the HVS enables us to develop computer models that can exploit features of the system. In this chapter, after introducing the structure of the HVS and some of its most important mechanisms, the visual attention process is described and a review of the use of these models in computer graphics is presented. Afterwards a discussion of some new new results in this area is given.

2 Human Visual System

The fundamental part of the HVS is the eye. It is an organ with approximately spherical shape [29], see Figure 1. The sphere has a radius of about 12 mm. In the protective envelope there are three pairs of extrinsic muscles that move the eye in its bony orbit. The eye consists of: cornea, pupil, lens, aqueous humour, vitreous body and retina.

The cornea is the outermost layer through which the external stimulus enters the eye. Although of a complex lamellar structure, the cornea is transparent and void of blood vessels. The pupil is the hole in the iris diaphram through which the light passes. The lens is a biconvex multilayered structure. The shape of the lens change during the accommodation and these changes occur mostly at its anterior surface, which touches the iris [29].

The aqueous humour is located between cornea and lens. This liquid, continuously generated and absorbed, controls the intraocular pressure, which is greater than the atmospheric pressure, to maintain the structural integrity of the eye. Between the lens and the retina, there is the vitreous body, which consists of a transparent jelly interlaced with fibers. The retina is a complex and multilayered structure lining most choroids, the vascular and pigmented layer attached to the sclera, the protecting envelope of the eye [29]. There are two elements of particular importance in the retina: fovea and photoreceptor. The fovea is a particular area of the retina where vision is most acute. There are two types of photo receptors in the retina: cones and rods. The rods are extremely sensitive to light and provide achromatic vision at scotopic levels of illumination raging from 10^{-6} to 10 cd/m^2 . The cones are less sensitive than the rods, but provide colour vision at photopic levels of illumination in the range of 0.01 to 10^8 cd/m^2. At light levels from 0.01 to 10 cd/m^2 both the rod and cone systems are active. This is known as the mesopic range [10].

Also in the fovea the cones photo receptors are presents, but they have a different structure than the cones in the retinal region. In the fovea there is the high density of cones, this gives to the fovea the exceptional capacity to resolve the fine details in an optical image focused there. The most central cones and each group of rods have a direct line to the brain

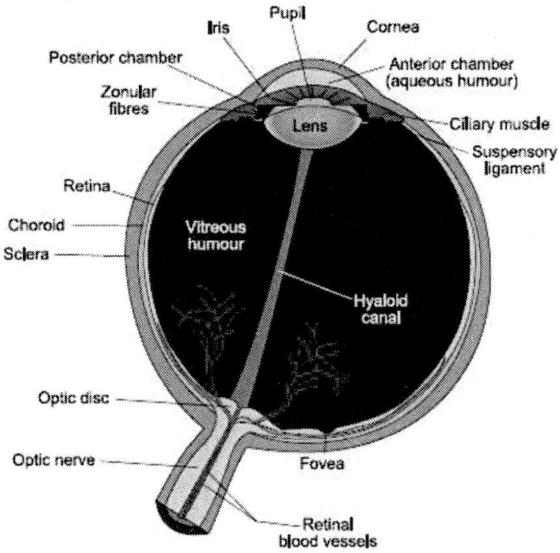

Figure 1: Human eye structure, after [33]

brain through the inner surface of the retina and the optic nerve. In addition to these direct connections there are myriads of local cross connections in the retina [20].

The formation image process in the HVS pipeline, is shown in Figure 2. The process can be divided in four stages: image formation, exposure control, detection and processing. The image formation is located in the cornea and the lens. Indeed the light reflected from an object strike the cornea and are thereby nearly focused on the retina. The lens completes the focusing. If there is a plenty of light, the iris diaphragm contracts so that the pupil become smaller and only the centre of the lens is used. This gives the sharpest image [20]. The radiant energy penetrating the cornea is not only brought to a sharp focus by the cornea and lens but is also modified in spectral composition by pigment, macula and lens, and transformed to nerve activity by pigments, rods and cones. Most of radiant energy is finally absorbed by pigment in the choroids coat. These patterns of nerve activity are propagated from the receptors to the brain [20]. There this information is elaborated and gives to the humans the capacity to see the image.

2.1 Human Visual Field and Eye Movements

The human $visual\ field$ can be separated in different areas where we have different levels of vision. The foveal vision, as reported in Section 2, has an area of approximately $2°$. The parafoveal vision has an area of about $20°$ and the perifoveal vision of about $50°$. Finally the peripheral vision occupies around $80°$ on both sides of the centre of attention [25].

The HVS uses six muscles to allow the eye to move with six degrees of human freedom. In using these muscles is able to provide five basic types of eye movements that allow to have the image always onto the foveal area. As reported in [32] these movement can be divided in two categories: $stabilising$ and $saccadic$ movements. The first one, is respon-

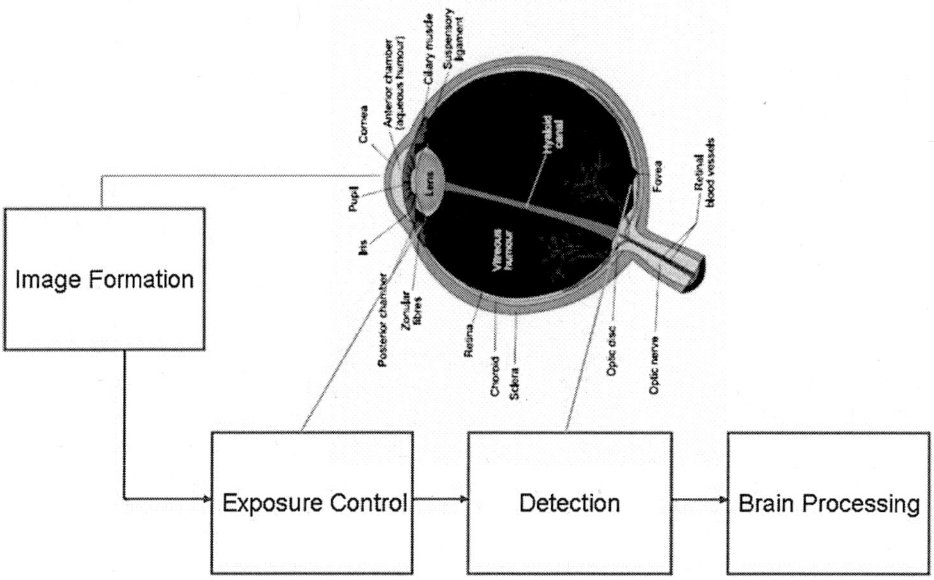

Figure 2: Pipeline of how the HVS reproduces the real image: red line is representing the output of each step of the pipeline, green line indicates where the step of the pipeline takes place in the eye structure.

sible for holding an image still on the retina. The second one, has the purpose of bringing objects of interest onto the fovea [25].

2.2 Visual Adaptation

The process by which the HVS adjusts itself to the conditions, under which the eyes are exposed to radiant energy, is called adaptation [20]. Adaptation is achieved through the coordinated action of mechanical, photochemical, and neural processes in the visual system. Adaptation can also be described through the physiological phenomenons happening inside the HVS. The HVS is able to work over a luminance range of nearly $14\ log$ units; despite the fact that the individual neural units, which make up the system, have a response range of only about $1.5\ log$ units [23]. With these mechanisms, the visual system moderates the effects of changing levels of illumination on visual response, providing sensitivity over a wide range of ambient light levels [10]. The pupil modifications in diameter according to the changes in luminance, as described in Section 2, produces about a log unit change in retinal luminance. This small change does not allow the pupil action to be sufficient to completely account for visual adaptation [23]. At high light intensities, the action of light depletes the photosensitive pigments in the rods and cones at a faster rate than chemical processes can restore them. This make the receptors less sensitive to light. This process is known as pigment bleaching [10]. The neural response produced by a photo receptor cell depends on chemical reactions produced by the action of light on the cell's photo pigments [Fe+96]. The cell's response to light is limited by the maximum rate and intensity of these chemical reactions. If the reactions are occurring near their maximum levels, and the amount of light striking the photo pigments is increased, the cell may not be able to fully signal the increase. This situation is know as saturation process [10]. The result of saturation is a response compression: above a certain level incremental increases in light intensity

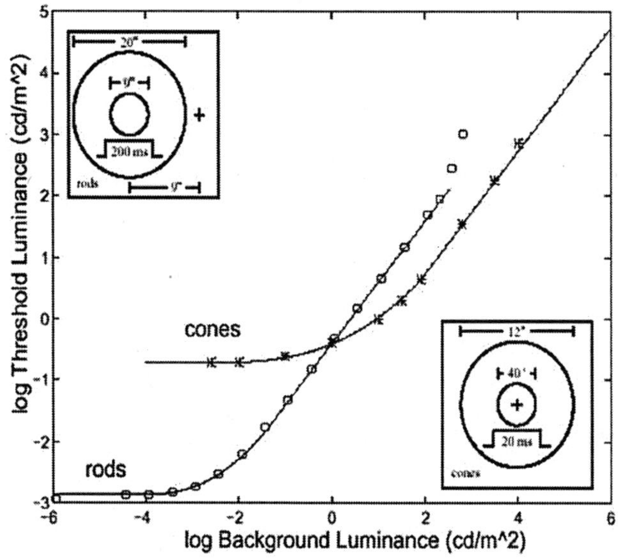

Figure 3: A psychophysical model of detection thresholds over the full range of vision (TVI), after [10].

will produce smaller and smaller changes in the cells response rate [10]. As described in Section 1.2, the rods and cone photo receptors are connected thought a network of neurons in the retina. Here an adaptive process that adjusts the base activity and gains the visual system to mitigate the effects of response compression in the photo receptors, takes place. These adaptive processes are subdivided in two classes: multiplicative and subtractive. The multiplicative process adjusts the gain of the system by effectively scaling the input by a constant related to the background luminance. This process acts very rapidly and accounts for changes in sensitivity over the first few seconds of adaptation [10]. A slower acting subtractive process reduces the base level of activity in the system caused by a constant background. This process accounts for the slow improvements in sensitivity measured over minutes of adaptation [1]. The action of these mechanisms is reflected in the changes in visibility, colour appearance, visual acuity, and sensitivity over the time, and can be observed in everyday experience and measured in psychophysical experiments [10]. A visual threshold is defined by the probability p of seeing a difference in brightness, hue, saturation, or a difference in some other attributes exhibited by given set of stimuli [29]. The effects of adaptation have been measured in threshold experiments. Figure 3 shows the results of a threshold experiment that measured the changes in visibility that occur with changes in the level of illumination [21]. These curves are known as $threshold - vs. - intensity$ (TVI) functions, and describe the dependence of the threshold from the background luminance. Over a wide range of background luminance, the size of the threshold increment increases in proportion to the background luminance making the functions linear on a $log - log$ scale. This linear relationship $\triangle L = kL$ is known as $Weber's$ law and indicates that the visual system has constant contrast sensitivity since the Weber contrast $\triangle L/L$ is constant over this range [21].

The most important kinds of adaptation are: dark, light and chromatic. The dark adaptation increases the visual sensitivity experienced when luminance level decreases. Light adaptation is the decrease in visual sensitivity upon increases in the overall level of illumination. The last important kind of visual adaptation is called chromatic adaptation. It is defined as the HVS capability to adjust to widely varying colours of illumination in order to approximately preserve the appearance of object colours [9]. The adaptation does not happen instantaneously, in fact it takes time. The time is not the same for all kinds of adaptation. Indeed, the time for dark adaptation is different than that for light adaptation.

3 Visual Attention

To understand complex scenes the HVS uses a process called visual attention. It allows the problem of understanding to be divided into a rapid series of computationally less demanding, localized visual analysis problems [13]. In other words, the HVS processes a complex scene by using shifting mechanisms that result in giving more attention to salient locations and less attention to unimportant regions. As reported in Section 2, the fovea provides the highest spatial and chromatic resolution than elsewhere in the retina. However the visual angle covered by the fovea is only approximately $2°$ and this makes the image, in our peripheral vison, perceived as unclear and blurred [4]. In order for the HVS to be able to capture detailed information from different areas of the visual environment the eyes do not scan the scene in a raster-like fashion, but rather they jump so that relevant objects fall sequentially on the fovea. This is known as saccade [30].

Purely related to the visual attention is the so called inattentional blindness. When attention is focused onto an item in a scene, details about the rest of the environment can literally go unnoticed. This is known as $Inattentional\ Blindness$ [16].

As defined in [19] the visual attention mechanisms comprises two different processes: $bottom - up$ and $top - down$.

3.1 Top-down Approach

The top-down process is driven by specific task that focuses the human observer's attention on a specific object relevant to the goal of the task. For exampple if the the goal is to take a pen on the desk, the human observer's attention will be concentrated on the desk area and in particular to the objects belong to this area and all the remaining objects in the scene will be completly ignored. This process is completly based on voluntary control; this means that even the objects that normally attract the observer's attention may be completly unoticed if they are irrelevant to the to the specific task [5]. Based on this characteristic the top-down process is often also called task-dependent. We may use this knowledge to build a $task\ map$ that defines the task objects within a scene which can predict the eye fixation points that scene. Taking the fixation points as the center of the visual angle of the fovea, the area belonging to this visual angle is the one where the human attention is focused [4].

3.2 Bottom-up Approach

The bottom-up process is purely stimulus driven in which the eyes are moved to specific details of the scene completly automatically. Consipicuous or salient stimuli include flickering in a static scene or very saturated colours, attracting involuntary and automatically attention.

These processes are independent from a specific task and operate very rapidly. The speed of this saliency-based form of attention is on the order of 25 to 50 ms per item [13]. In other words the bottom-up process is attracted involuntary by saliency stimuli in the scene and it is also called image-based saliency. Using this knowledge we can compute a *saliency map* that is a two dimensional topographical map that encodes saliency, at every location of the visual scene. The saliency map receives inputs from early visual processing, and provide an efficient control strategy in which the focus of attention simply scans the saliency map in order of decreasing saliency [13]. Any model of bottom-up attention is costituted by five components: early visual futures computation, their integration, generation of attentional scanpaths, the interaction between the expression of attention with (*overt* attention) and without (*covert* attention) eye movements and finally, the interplay between attention and scene understanding. The early visual futures are computed across the entire visual scene, and their integration will yield a single attentional control command [13].

4 Visual Attention in Computer Graphics

The physically and perceptually accurate simulation of the real world on computers is playing key role in many major applications, including training, design and visualisation. However, for such applications, it is essential that these highly realistic, environments are generated in real time, allowing users to interact with the virtual world in a seamless manner. The current state-of-the-art high fidelity virtual reality may take many seconds to compute on even high performance computers, while real-time systems accept a severe reduction in quality as the trade-off to achieving interactive rates.

In the last twenty years researcher in computer graphics have started to take advantage of visual perceptions aspects of the HVS for reducing the computational costs of complex rendering techniques. Part of this work attempts to develop high level of models of the HVS that incorporate the spatial process and sensitivity changes behaviours [2], and also the visual masking mechanism [11]. Others make use of perceptual metrics [17] [3] [22] [18] [26] [8]. Renedring large scale geometric dataset at interactive rates is also a big challenge in computer graphics. In this field of research Luebke et al. [14] use aspectcs of visual perception to reduce level of detail and thus the computational costs. Furthermore visual perception aspects of the HVS have been used to evaluate the perceptually fidelity of images [7].

Recently visual attention approaches have been explored in order to accelerate the computational time required for complex rendering algorithms such as global illumination techniques. In this Section we will review the work that make use of visual attention model in the computer graphics context.

The bottom-up (known as saliency map [12] [31]) and top-down (known as task map [6]) visual attention processes has been used to significantly reduce the computation of high-fidelity global illumination calculations. Sundstedt et al. [26] combined both saliency and task maps into a single Importnace Map to further reduce overall computation time in image rendering while preserving the perceptual quality of the image. In addition, Longhurst et al. [15] developed an hardware implementation of the bottom-up model presented by Itti et al. [13] for developing a saliency map for interactive applications. Also *inattentional blindness* has been investigated in Cater et al. [5]. Inattentional blindness [16] is when the attention is focused onto an item in a scene, details about the rest of teh environment, such as lighting, resolution, level of detail and even the presence/absence of objects can go unoticed [4]. In Cater et al. [5] a series of experiments with 160 subjects were conducted in order to verify the behaviour of inattentional blindness in computer graphics context. They discovered that 90% of the subjects were unable to recall the correct details of some objects in the visual scene when they were concentrated on another task.

4.1 Recent Results

In this Section we will show some recent results obtained in the *High Dynamic Range Imaging* (HDR) area for real-time applications. HDR is becoming very popular area and a large range of applications, outside of computer graphics, are starting to make use of it. This technology is able to capture the luminance dynamic range available in the real world. However, the accurate simulation of the distribution of light energy in scenes does not guarantee that images generated from this simulation will have a realistic visual appearance. The main reasons for this are: first, the dynamic range of the light energy in the scene may be vastly different from the dynamic range that can be produced by the display device. In fact, the current output display devices such as projectors or screens, have several technological limitations, for example; limited colour gamut and contrast, low dynamic range, limited spatial resolution, (usually) limited field of view, and non trivial workarounds to achieve stereo capacity. it is necessary to simulate the behaviour of the HVS to capture the correct appearance of the original scene. For example, the viewing conditions of the two observers (scene and display) may be completely different. The conversion from the HDR to display luminance is known as $Tone - Mapping$ (TM). TM is a very important last step in the (re-)production of realistic images and several operators have been proposed, but is still prohibitive to have a complex TM operator that produce high quality results in real-time. We have make use of visual attention models to accelerate the computational costs rerquired to compute complex high quality TM operators.

From our preliminary experiments we discovered that an edge detector such as the *Canny* model is able to capture enough information and the saliency map build with this information ($C - Map$) is comparable with the saliency map obtained with a more sophisticated visual attention model ($V - Map$) such as [12]. To demonstrate this we have compared the two tone mapped images, obtained using the two different saliency maps, with the ground truth tone mapped image ($G - T$) that does not make use of saliency information.

To perform these tests we have used two well known quality metrics: *Visual Difference Predictor* (VDP) [27] and *Structural Similarity Index* ($SSIM$) [28], on several HDR images. The VDP gives as output a percentage of pixels that are perceivably different by the HVS [27]. Our HVS has the property to highly adapt to extract structural information from the viewing field. Based on this concept, a measure of structural information changes provides a good approximation to perceive image distortion [28]. The $SSIM$ index provides a measure of the structural information changes in the image. In other words, it indicates the degree of similarities between two images: 1 perfect similarity and 0 completely different. The images used in the experiments are shown in Figure 4.

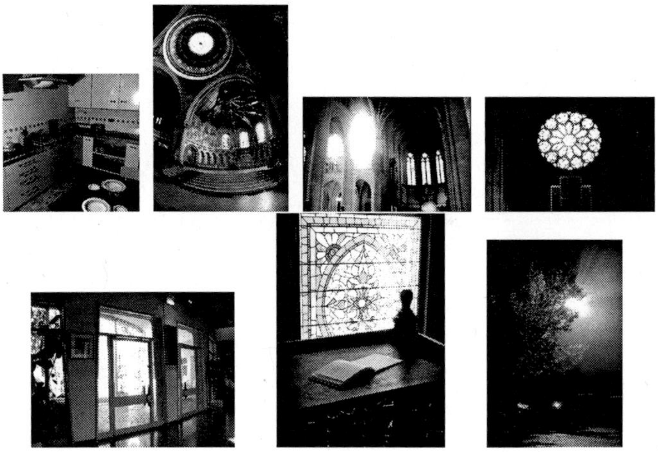

Figure 4: Images used in the experiments: form the left (Image 1) to the right of the second row (Image 7).

Table 1: Results of the quality comparison using the VDP metric, for comparing the output obtained with the C-Map and the V-Map vs. the output obtained with the G-T. The VDP metric gives the percentage of pixels that are perceived different by the HVS.

HDR Images	C-Map vs G-T	V-Map vs G-T
Image 1	0.04	0.07
Image 2	2.41	3.62
Image 3	1.47	2.81
Image 4	0.38	0.09
Image 5	0.21	0.35
Image 6	2.72	2.05
Image 7	0.07	0.18

From the results shown in Table 1, the images obtained using the two different maps ($C - Map$ and $V - Map$) are not perceived by the HVS as different. In most of the cases the performances obtained with the $C - Map$ are better than the one obtained with the visual attention model. In fact the VDP detected a small percentage of pixels perceived as different for the output obtained with the $C - Map$. This can be explained observing the saliency maps build with $Canny$ edge detector and the visual attention model (Figure 5).

The two output maps are quite similar and the $V - Map$ is identfying redundant saliency areas that do not add any quality improvement in the final tone mapped output image. Figure 6 and Figure 7 show images obtained using the $C - Map$ (left), the image obtained with the $G - T$ (center) and the VDP map showing the pixels (red dots) perceived as different by the HVS, superimposed on the $C - Map$ (right). It is difficult to notice strong differences between the two images obtained using the two different maps, and this is confirmed by the VDP map where few pixels are shown as perceived different by the

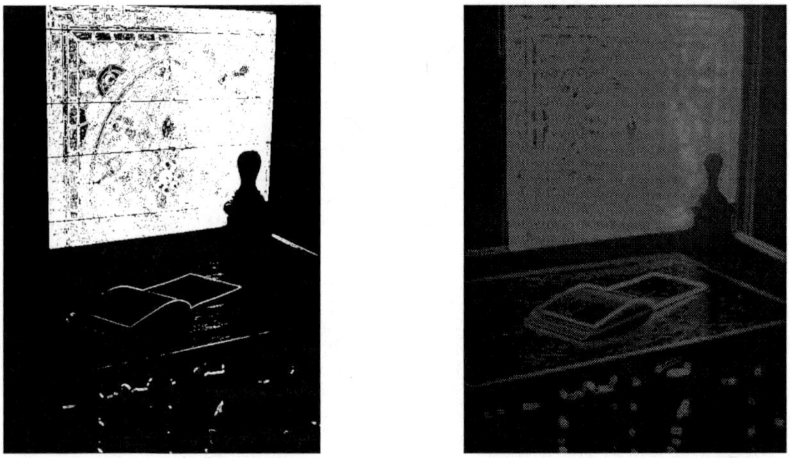

Figure 5: Saliency mas: (left) C-Map (right) V-Map. In the V-Map we have different levels of gray that for our application will be transformed in a unique gray level making it similar to the C-Map.

HVS. In our opinion the $V-Map$ is capturing saliency areas that are going to unnoticed by the HVS. We need to identify the high contrast edges, that are identified by transition areas between regions with strong changes in the luminance level. It seems that an edge detector is able to give a strong response near foreground/background silhouettes and in textured regions, identifying the saliency areas that are going to be noticed by the HVS. This phenomenon is even more evident in real-time context such as video applications where several frames, representing the visual scene (usually 25-30 frame per second fps), are processed and these more details identified by the complex viusal attention model may be completly unoticed by the HVS. The final experiment we performed was to confirm the quality obtained with $C - Map$ using the $SSIM$ metric (see Table 2).

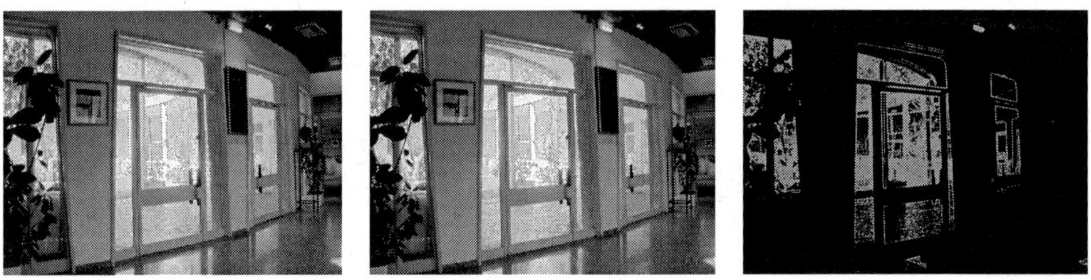

Figure 6: Quality comparison between the images obtained using the C-Map (left) and the ground truth (center). The VDP map (right) shows the pixels perceived as different by the HVS (red dots) superimposed on the C-Map. Belgium image courtesy of Dani Lischinski.

Also, the $SSIM$ metric confirms the results of the VDP metric; the two images are practically similar.

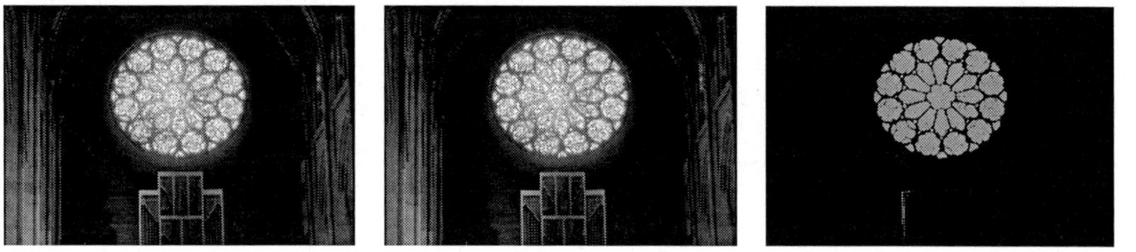

Figure 7: Quality comparison between the images obtained using the $C\text{-}Map$ (left) and the ground truth (center). The VDP map (right) shows the pixels perceived as different by the HVS (red dots) superimposed on the $C\text{-}Map$. Rosette image courtesy of Paul Debevec.

Table 2: Results of the quality comparison using the $SSIM$ metric. We compared the output obtained with the use of the $C\text{-}Map$ vs. the gorund trouth $G\text{-}T$.

HDR Images	C-Map vs. G-T
Image 1	0.9968
Image 2	0.9876
Image 3	0.9761
Image 4	0.9982
Image 5	0.9853
Image 6	0.9925
Image 7	0.9972

5 Conclusions and Future Work

We have shown how in computer graphics applications such as the tone mapping, the saliency map developed making use of sophisticated visual attention models is capturing information that often does not add any quality improvement to the output image. On the other hand, the detection of this additional information drastically increases the computation time of the saliency map preventing the use of these shopisticated visual attention model in real-time applications. From these preliminary results a number of questions arises: Are the visual attention mechanisms of the HVS different, in term of complexity, within the visual experience of the observer? In other words, based on the visual experience of the observer can we use different level of complexity degree of visual attention model for capturing properly the saliency information? Are these mechanisms different in case of dynamic environment? In fact all research on the development of visual attention models is based on the analysis of still images and not on a continuose stream of different frames such as video. This introduces different complexity to the problem and as consequence different visual attention model may need to be developed. Future work should investigate these results in more detail and based on them develop a more appropriated salinecy map for real-time applications.

References

[1] E.H. Adelson, *Saturation and adaptation in the rod system.* Vision Research, Volume **22**, pp. 1299-1312 (1982).

[2] M. Bolin and G. Meyer, *A frequency based ray tracer.* In SIGGRAPH Conference Proceedings, pp. 409418 (1995).

[3] M.R. Bolin and G.W. Meyer, *A Perceptually based adaptive sampling algorithm.* Computer Graphics, 32(Annual Conference Series), pp. 299-309 (1998).

[4] A. Chalmers, K. Cater and D. Mafioli, *Visual Attention Models for Producing High Fidelity Graphics Efficiently.* Spring Conference on Computer Graphics SCCG (2003).

[5] K. Cater, A. Chalmers and P. Ledda, *Selective quality rendering by exploiting human inattentional blindness: looking but not seeing.* In Proceedings of the ACM Symposium on Virtual reality software and technology, pp. 1724 (2002).

[6] K. Cater, A. Chalmers and G. Ward, *Detail to Attention:Exploiting Visual Tasks for Selective Rendering.* In Proceedings of the Eurographics Symposium on Rendering, pp. 270280 (2003).

[7] S. Daly, *The Visible Differences Predictor: an algorithm for the assessment of image fidelity.* Digital Image and Human Vision, pp.189-206 (1993).

[8] R. Dumont, F. Pellacini and J. A. Ferwerda, *Perceptually driven decision theory for interactive realistic rendering.* ACM Trans. Graph. Volme **22** (2) pp. 151181 (2003).

[9] M. D. Fairchild, *Colour Appearance Models.* Addison Wesley (1998).

[10] J. A. Ferwerda, S. N. Pattanaik, P. Shirley, and D. P. Greenberg, *A Model of Visual Adaptation for Realistic Image Synthesis.* ACM Computer Graphics (Proc. of SIGGRAPH), pp. 249-258 (1996).

[11] J. A. Ferwerda, S. N. Pattanaik, P. Shirley, and D. P. Greenberg, *A model of visual masking for computer graphics* In SIGGRAPH Conference Proceedings, pp. 143152 (1997).

[12] L. Itti and C. Koch and E. Niebur, *A model of saliency based visual attention for rapid scene analysis.* Pattern Analysis and Machine Intelligence, Volume **20**, pp. 1254-1259 (1998).

[13] L. Itti and C. Koch, *Computational Modelling of Visual Attention.* Nature Review Neuroscience, Volume **2** (2001).

[14] D. Lubeke and B. Hallen, *Perceptually driven simplification for interactive rendering.* In Proceedings of 12th Eurographics Workshop on Rendering, pp. 221-223 (2001).

[15] P. Longhur(st, K. Debattista and A. Chalmers, *GPU Based Saliency Map for High-Fidelity Selective Rendering.* In Afrigraph Conference Proceedings, (2006).

[16] A. Mack and I. Rock, *Inattentional Blindness.* Proceedings of Symposium on Interactive 3D Graphics, Massachusetts Institute of Technology Press (1998).

[17] K. Myszkowski, *The Visible Difference Predictor: Application to Global illumination Problems.* Proceeding of Eurographics Workshop on Rendering, G. Drettakis and N. Max Eds., pp. 223-236 (1998).

[18] K. Myszkowski, *Perception-based global illumination, rendering, and animation techniques.* In Proceedings of the 18th spring conference on Computer graphics ACM, pp. 1324 (2002).

[19] W. James, *A saliency-based search mechanism for overt and covert shifts of visual attention* Principles of Psychology, New York: Holt (1890).

[20] D. B. Judd, and G. Wyszecki, *Colour in Business, Science and Industry.* Jhon Wiley adn Sons, 3nd Edition, 1975.

[21] S. N. Pattanaik, J. A. Ferwerda, M. Fairchild, and D. P. Greenberg, *A Multiscale Model of Adaptation and Spatial Vision for Realistic Image Display.* , ACM Computer Graphics (Proc. of SIGGRAPH), pp. 287–298 (1998).

[22] M. Ramasubramanian, S. N. Pattanaik, and D. P. Greenberg, *A perceptually Based Physical Error Metric for Realistic Image Synthesis.* , In Proceedings of the 26th Annual Conference on Computer Graphics and Interactive Techniques, ACM Press/Addison-Wesley Publishing Co., pp. 73-82 (1999).

[23] L. Spillman, and J.S. Werner, *Visual perception: the neurophysiological foundations.* San Diego Accademic press 1990.

[24] D. Simons and C. Chabris, *Gorillas in our midst: Sustained inattentional blindness for dynamic events.* Perception, Volume **28**, pp. 1059-1074 (1999).

[25] V. Sundstedt, *Rendering and Validation of High-Fidelity Graphics using Region-of-Interest.* PhD Thesis Bristol University UK (2007).

[26] V. Sundstedt, A. Chalmers, K. Cater and K. Debattista, *Top-Down Visual Attention for Efficient Rendering of Task Related Scenes.* VMV 2004 - Vision, Modelling and Visualization (2004).

[27] Author, *Available software, Visible Difference Predictor at MPI Max Planck Institute,* **url:**http://www.mpi-inf.mpg.de/resources/hdr/vdp/.

[28] Z. Wang and A. C. Bovik and H. R. Sheikh and E. P. Simoncelli, *Image quality Assesment: From error visibility to structural similarity* IEEE Transaction on Image Processing, Volume **13**, number 4 (2004).

[29] G. Wyszecki, and W. S. Stiles, *Color Science: Concepts and Methods, Quantitative Data and Formulae.* Jhon Wiley adn Sons, 2nd Edition, (1982).

[30] A. Yarbus, *Eye movements during perception of complex objects.* In Eye Movements and Vision, pp. 171196 (1967).

[31] H. Yee and S. Pattanaik and D.P. Greenberg, *Spatiotemporal Sensitivity and Visual Attention for Efficient Rendering of Dynamic Environments.* ACM Transaction on Computer Graphics, Voume **20** (1), pp. 39-65 (2001).

[32] K. Lukander, *Mobile usability: Measuring Gaze Point on Handheld Devices.* Masters thesis, Helsinki University of Technology (2003).

[33] Wikipedia. http://www.wikipedia.org.

INDEX

D

E

F

O

P

Q

R